Crazy, Chronic Life: A Handbook

To all the members of Chronic Illness Support for Crazy, Chronic Lives-
your love and support made this possible

Table of Contents

Foreword..1
Crazy, Chronic Guide to Common Chronic Illness Symptoms..........3
Battling Brain Fog 5
Fighting Fatigue..18
Chronic Pain 30
Bodily Fluids, Functions, and General Funk.........................42
Crazy, Chronic Survival Guide for Doctor's Appointments 52
Becoming a 55
What to do when you can't do anything...............................65
Crazy, Chronic Survival Guide to Packing and Road Trips............75
Accepting Disabled Life..81
A Day in the Chronic Life 91
Crazy, Chronic Survival Guide to Holidays and Family Events 102
Friendships and Chronic Illness- It's possible to have both. 106
Crazy, Chronic Survival Guide to Hanging Out with Healthy Friends
....117
On Faith and Healing...120
Crazy, Chronic Survival Guide- Going to Church 131
Crazy Chronic Survival Guide- Surviving a Lifelong Diagnosis...136
Getting a Diagnosis- AKA The Long and Lonely Road 140
Research, Awareness, and Advocacy....................................150
Victim vs. Advocate 162
Body Image and Illness- I make broken look good....................172
Caregivers as Romantic Partners..183
When the Normally Healthy Partner is Sick- AKA The Grand
Apocalypse 193
Medical Anxiety- AKA Meltdowns of Epic Proportions..............200
Letters to Those Who Don't Understand................................207
Dear Church,..208
Dear Mean Mugger,...210
Dear hotel staff, ...212
Dear Social Media Merchant,...214

Foreword

Marriage is a cooperative process, and Tiffany and I are the ultimate team. In almost all aspects of life, we do everything together. We genuinely enjoy each other's company. Some of these things we share are great like Disney World, concerts, vacations, and travelling. Other aspects are more difficult. Without getting into details that come out in the chapters to follow, I will just say that Tiffany has a chronic disease. Some days are tough and some days aren't so bad, but anyone without a chronic disease would still call them bad days. Though Tiffany carries the actual pain of her disease, I'm still a part of the marriage and I do what I can to alleviate it and keep her spirits up.

This book is another joint Early endeavor. Most of the fun, pain, anxiety, and silliness that follow were shared experiences, so we decided we should write this book together. Basically, the book's development occurred over cooking dinner. While Tiffany works on dinner, we talk about our day and recent events. Mine dealt with work and all the things it entails. Very often it was rote and rarely involved any physical pain other than when I busted my nose on a door. Tiffany's day was often very different. Her joints had popped out, she had terrible headaches, bad doctor's visits, and most of all her worries about the future. Many nights

1

she mentioned she wished there was a "How To" book to better prepare her for some of the thing that she faced. We looked on Amazon and there were not very many helpful books. I mean, there were some books, but basically, they dealt with dealing with the fact you have a chronic disease rather how to still enjoy your life with it. I remember being surprised because there are books on every subject under the sun. We thought we should fix this problem. We realized that others could learn from our victories and defeats by writing down some of the best stories, lessons learned, and problems encountered, in the hopes it would help some other person whose life has dealt a similar hand.

Over a two-year period, Tiffany and I talked about places we had been (football games, doctors' visits, family events, etc.), and she told me what problems she faced that day and I made notes. Later, I put them down into a rough draft. Tiffany took my rough draft, added her own turn of phrase, light-hearted stories, and personal flair. Basically, I was the grunt work, and she was the vision. I hope you find this book helpful, and it gives you some ideas about how to enjoy life with the problems your body carries.

Joe

Crazy, Chronic Guide to Common Chronic Illness Symptoms

Symptoms. *Everything* is a symptom in my life. Some come and go; others take up residence and become a permanent part of me. My body is one big party with a lot of unwanted guests- like fatigue and pain and bladder dysfunction. Are we having fun yet? Has anyone else noticed that this party stinks?

Obviously, we all suffer. That's why it's called a chronic illness and not a chronic birthday party. However, our illnesses are as varied as we are. We have a myriad of symptoms that complicate our days, and I won't even pretend to understand the depth of suffering any other person has endured. Having said that, there are a few symptoms that are common among our chronically ill tribe. These are the symptoms I see discussed daily on social media forums. These are the things we all "get." If I tell a fellow crazy, chronic friend that my fatigue is crushing me, he or she will understand that I am *not* simply saying that I'm tired. So, even though I *know* that we all understand what these symptoms are and how they affect us personally, I want them explained. I want to find a way to explain

3

to my husband or my family or a friend what I am actually feeling. I want all of us to have a resource to help us describe and manage what is happening in our bodies as well as possible.

For that reason, I have dedicated a section of this book to our most common symptoms. Each chapter in this section will tackle a symptom (or a conglomeration of symptoms) to tell what it is, how we are affected, and how to deal with it as well as possible. Do I have all the answers? Nope, of course not. Do I have enough experience to start a discussion? Sure. We all do. That's what makes us all part of this crazy, chronic party that none of us actually wanted to attend.

So, here it is, the Crazy, Chronic Guide to Brain fog, Fatigue, Pain, and General Bodily Funk . . .

Battling Brain Fog

Brain fog is such a lame term. It sounds like something you make up when you're called on to answer a question in class and you're totally unprepared. ("Uh . . . I'm sorry, Teacher. My brain feels so foggy.") It sounds like a byproduct of recreational pharmaceuticals. However, it is a totally legit term used to describe "symptoms of confusion, forgetfulness, and lack of focus and mental clarity." (bebrainfit.com) In other words, it is a real thing that happens and is described by patients and physicians alike.

Having said that, brain fog is *not* a medically recognized diagnosis. You'll never be officially diagnosed with brain fog, because brain fog isn't an actual disease or disorder. It's a symptom of a disease or disorder. It can happen for many different reasons. For example, some medications can cause confusion or impaired thinking (and, really, nothing thrills me more than a medicine that will clear up my eczema but make me a babbling idiot- *eye roll*). Others experience brain fog because their pain or fatigue (or an awful combination of the two) make them so distracted they can't focus. Still, others have cognitive struggles for physiological reasons. For example, my friends with dysautonomia (including me) have impaired thought and reasoning because of their bodies' inability to pump blood to their brains. Others have difficulty thinking because of neurological deficits, chemical imbalances, or deteriorating brain pathways. For most of us, it's probably a frustrating combination of all the above. Regardless of the reason, the majority of us dealing with chronic illness are stuck on the struggle bus when life requires quick recall or decision-making.

Imagine trying to drink a delicious beverage (Southern US friends, let's imagine that beverage is a sweet tea. Yummmm!), but there is a hole in your straw. No matter how hard you try, you cannot overcome the straw's gaping defect in order to adequately enjoy your drink. You might get occasional sputters of liquid, but there's never enough to satisfy you. That, my friends, is how brain fog makes me feel. I feel like my brain just won't connect. I'm trying, but nothing is happening. My brain is using maximum effort in order to produce minimal (and disappointing) cognitive output. I have literally given myself a headache trying to remember the most banal words.

When this happens (and it happens a lot), I feel so embarrassed and frustrated. I mean, seriously? Am I really this dumb? Did I forget how to "human" again? And then, the emotions hit. For me, if I'm frustrated, I cry. It's not a sadness cry; it's a "I can't even handle my life at this moment" cry. I'm pretty sure that when I'm babbling incoherently then bursting into tears people are wondering what the heck my problem is. I feel like I should wear a sign that says, "I swear, I'm not on drugs. My brain only functions under specific conditions which are unknown even to me."

Chronic illness is hard enough. My body is rebelling day in and day out. I don't need embarrassment and shame to go along with my array of other issues. This is the aggravation of chronic illness for me. It's not just my symptoms- although they're certainly bad enough. It's the range of feelings and emotions that go along with the symptoms. Seriously, body, it's bad enough that you don't function correctly, but if you could refrain from making me feel like a general failure at life that'd be great.

If you've ever had to deal with a really difficult or unpleasant person, you know that you need a plan to handle the madness and preserve your own sanity. Dealing with brain fog is similar. It will always be frustrating. I will always be embarrassed when I'm stumbling over words or forgetting how to tie my shoes, but there are things I can do to make handling brain fog easier.

1. Think first- act second.

This does not come naturally to me. I tend to blurt out whatever crosses my foggy mind and pay the price later. I have a gift for confusing or offending those around me with a single unplanned statement. However, when the stakes are high (speaking in public, making an appointment, introducing myself), I try to make a plan before I speak. I'll think about exactly what I need to say. I'll make a mental list of key words I'll need (If I don't, simple words like "paper" or "olives" will completely escape me).

True story- the other day I told my husband I needed him to open the jar of "pickle dots" for me. I meant olives. I just didn't find the word before I spoke. Joe is used to this lunacy, and we laugh at my odd word choice and proceed. In any other setting, I would need to ensure that I knew the name of whatever salty deliciousness was in the jar before I asked for help with it.

There have actually been times when I've assigned a keyword to each of my fingers. (I know, I sound insane, but stay with me here.) For example, if I need to ask the hotel desk clerk for more towels, I will find 3 key words that will be needed to make my request.

1. Room number

2. Towels

3. Please

Then, when I actually go to the desk, I will discretely hold up a finger for each number to ensure that I've said everything I intended. "I'm in (1) room 224, and I need more (2) towels, (3) please." Is that way too complicated for simply asking for towels? Yes, absolutely. Is it sometimes necessary to ensure that I carry out the necessary plan? Yes, absolutely. If I don't have a plan in place, there's a very real possibility that I'll end up saying something awkward. "Hi, I'm in a room, and I need to be dried." Ugh.

2. Make lists- all the lists.

If I absolutely must accomplish something during the day, I had better make a list. If I have to accomplish multiple things, I should make a list of all the lists I need to complete. I'm serious. If you're brain is a foggy mess like mine, don't assume you'll remember anything. Don't take for granted that you will remember to put gas in the car when you see the "Empty" light illuminated. Put it on the list. Don't have the audacity to believe that you will remember to fix dinner just because you fix dinner every single night. I'm serious. Put. It. On. A. List. Use all the lists. Cross each item off the list as you complete it. Never cross an item off the list as you're beginning to do it. You might stop before you accomplish the task. I can't begin to explain how many times I've looked at my grocery list in the grocery store, crossed off an item as I started to pick it up, then got completely distracted before I could actually retrieve the item. (It's a little inconvenient, but I've learned how to make a lot of recipes minus the key ingredient. Brain fog has made me resourceful anyway.)

I have a tendency to make a list and then leave it at home. (And my dog never answers when I call to ask her to read it to me!) Now, after I make a list, I take a picture of it with my phone. That way, if I lose or forget the list, there's a backup copy. (It's also really handy in case my husband offers to run my errands for me- which is the best case scenario.)

3. Plan an escape route.

Life isn't always polite enough to give you an abscond when your brain is failing to function properly. It's just not socially acceptable to cower under a blanket in a fetal position every time I embarrass myself. (I'm a hot mess. I would basically never leave the protection of a blanket if I did this.) However, I plan an escape when possible. Typically, I use words as my escape. For example, if my brain is fading fast, I have the following statement memorized- "Sorry. My brain is tired. I'll e-mail you about this later." Is it rude? I don't know- maybe a little, but it's kinder to everyone involved (including me) than me being reduced to tears while mumbling incoherently. That statement has saved me on occasions when the present conversation or activity wasn't on that day's list.

I have the tendency to tell long, rambling stories that may or may not have an actual point. (I'm a blast at a party. Can't you tell?) A college friend told me once that when you're telling a story and realize it's going absolutely nowhere, say, "And then I found five dollars!" You know what? It works! No matter who you're talking to (or rambling at, in my case), if you tell them you found five dollars, they'll say, "Wow! That's great!" It's the ultimate story saver.

*Note: Use the five dollar trick with caution. Some friends will ask to borrow the hypothetical $5, and the situation will become more awkward.

If you have no words left to even attempt to get out of the conversation, tie your shoe. It sounds ridiculous, but it works. It'll provide you a few seconds to gather your thoughts, and sometimes the change in position helps (or you could faint- which is the ultimate conversation killer). I've "tied my shoes" only to realize my shoes didn't have shoestrings before. No one noticed or if they did, they were kind enough not to comment.

4. Written communication is always better.

I've said (somewhat jokingly) for years that phone calls require too much commitment for me. If I call you, I have to ask how you're doing. Listen to your stories. Then, I have to remember the reason I called and actually have that conversation. Don't get me wrong- it's not that I don't *want* to talk to you. I probably do. But if I call you with a purpose, I don't want to be deterred by formalities. I will forget why I called. That's why I prefer written communication. If it's an option, I will always text or e-mail.

Written communication is easier to refer back to if you forget what someone said. Have you ever hung up with Aunt Wanda after discussing Thanksgiving dinner assignments and forgot what you told her you would contribute to the meal? Yeah, me too. (Always bring a dessert. People will forgive you for forgetting the turkey if you bring a delicious pie. I promise.) If you text or e-mail, you can re-read the conversation. It's a life saver. I don't always remember what I've read, but words typically don't go anywhere (Thank goodness my e-mail saves deleted mail!), so I can look up the needed information anytime.

There's ample time to think about what you're saying when you're writing. You're typically not rushed when you're writing/ typing what you have to say. You can be more clear and specific when you write. I have lost count of how many times I have spoken to someone only to have her reply, "I have no clue what you just said." It's not that this Kentucky girl's hillbilly dialect is *that* hard to understand (although it is an acquired skill). It's that I'm trying to get words out too quickly. I don't mean to jabber at you; it just happens. Writing/ typing/ texting requires me to slow down and articulate my thoughts. I know, beyond a shadow of a doubt, that I communicate better through written language. If I write I'm typically able to communicate while I'm comfortable and working on my own schedule. Trust me- I sound much smarter under those circumstances.

It's probably best to explain to those closest to you that written communication is easier for you. We live in a time dominated by text and e-mail, so most people won't think much of it. However, I'm finding that everything in life is less complicated if I communicate my needs to others.

(Of course, there's a chance that written communication doesn't work best for you, and that's perfectly fine. It's helpful to me, and it makes sense based on my needs. If it doesn't work for you, well, that's just further illustration of the varied needs among my chronic illness family.)

5. If the conversation is very important, bring a less foggy brain with you.

There are times when it is especially inconvenient to have a brain that feels like it's made of oatmeal. I have no clue how many doctors' appointments I've attended only to realize afterward that I had absolutely no memory of what happened during the appointment (which, depending on the doctor, is sometimes a blessing). I've learned that for all things medical, legal, or professional, I need to bring a backup brain. Ask a spouse, friend, or family member to accompany you to important meetings or appointments. Ask your backup brain to make notes of important things that you hear during the appointment. Of course, you should also take notes, but now you will have someone's notes to compare to yours. (I've found that people will do nearly anything if you promise to buy them lunch afterward. It's possible, however, that I just have exceptionally hungry friends.)

If you can't find someone to attend an appointment with you- or if the nature of the appointment is too confidential to invite someone else to join you, consider using a voice recorder. (There are several free apps that will allow you to do this through your phone.) Always ask any other people in the meeting if it's okay if you record them. If you're going to the meeting alone, it might be a good idea to call the office beforehand and ask if you can record the appointment. Some people may not be comfortable being recorded, and while that is certainly their right, you might want to reschedule for a time when someone can accompany you.

Lastly, bring a list with you. (Can you tell that I really love lists?) Bring a list of questions you want to discuss. (Jot down the answers if you're not recording the meeting.) I typically write more questions than I actually plan to ask. I put the most pressing questions at the top of my list. If I make it through those questions with time to spare, then I move on to the less significant questions. This helps me keep the appointment moving in a direction that is most helpful to me. It also ensures that I will stay focused. There's nothing worse than realizing you spent time (and typically money) by discussing something that had no significant value to your well-being. Brain fog fail.

6. Give yourself a break.

Guess what? If you follow every single rule as though I've written commandments just for you, you'll still have brain fog fails. It just happens. You can put a plan into place; you can even have a safety net, but sometimes you will still swing and miss. It's okay. Laugh it off; roll your eyes; smile really big, or find five dollars. However you handle the situation is the right way to handle it. I've used the wrong words (I swear, my mouth is like a bad autocorrect program!); I've tripped over my feet; I've failed to recognize people that I should know, and I've thought I recognized people I've never seen before. You know what? I haven't died from embarrassment yet. (Although, I may have gotten close a time or two.) Brain fog can be embarrassing, and embarrassment can be debilitating. We have too many other issues, however, to let embarrassment be the thing that keeps us from enjoying life. Smile, laugh, shrug, but just keep doing your best. You're sick, and life is complicated. But . . . here you are, trying to function. You're doing great; I promise. Nothing is going to stop you- not even a brain that feels like it's made of oatmeal.

Fighting Fatigue

It's not lost on me that even as I'm beginning this chapter I am struggling to keep my eyes open. My muscles are aching from exertion, and all I've done today is look at a computer screen. The struggle is real, friends. Chronic fatigue is described as "prolonged fatigue not relieved by rest" (the-medicaldictionary.com), but even that is not the most accurate description. Chronic fatigue is always feeling tired to the bone. It's the type of tired that goes far beyond "sleepy" and actually aches. No matter where I'm at- any given time of the day- I'm always aware that more than anything I would really like to lie down.

At this point, my fatigue is so much a part of who I am that I cannot tell what is a part of my personality and what is a part of my chronic illness. I typically have no clue if I'm exhausted or socially unambitious (although I have a suspicion that both are factors). I have become such an introvert as I've gotten older that I make trips to the restroom when I'm around people just to get a break from all the socializing. I can't decide if I actually like time alone that much or if I just long for time to rest. As much as I want to say that chronic illness does not define me, there are times when my personality can be summed up by "fatigued."

I've fallen asleep basically everywhere I've been at one point or the other. I've slept in movie theaters, rides at Disney World (I feel like I could write a guide about the best rides to nap on in Disney.), at restaurant tables, and in my car- sitting in the driver's seat (learning experience). I can and do sleep everywhere. Once, Joe and I were eating lunch at a packed restaurant before a University of Tennessee football game. I was so painfully tired that I truly couldn't hold my head up, so I told Joe I needed a "5 second nap". A 5 second nap is when I lay my head down while Joe slowly counts to 5 (which typically takes around 20 seconds, because he's considerate- not because he's a slow counter). Then I pick my head back up or else I would be a disgusting, drooling mess. During my 5 seconds of slumber, a fellow fan walked by, smacked the table, and yelled, "This one partied too hard last night!" Ugh. Just ugh. That's right, buddy. I slept 13 hours last night, and I'm still wrecked. Party freakin time, dude.

My exhaustion affects everything I do. It's impossible to make plans. Well, technically, I make a lot of plans; the follow through is the impossible part. I *want* to go to the movies with you. I would *love* to check out your

19

new book club. But, to be honest, I have no idea if I'll even have the energy to put on respectable pants. It's hard to be a good friend- or even make new friends- when you really don't feel like doing anything- ever. I'm 31 years old. Most of my friends have kids of their own and do fun things like meet friends and have a group outing to the park. Me? I want a group nap- kids optional.

If I'm being entirely honest, though, no one really cares that I'm tired. I don't mean that in a self-victimizing way either. We live in a culture that equates fatigue with laziness. They're very different. As a matter of fact, if I would just be lazy, my fatigue would probably not be so intense. Since society doesn't grant me a pass on adulting just because I have a chronic illness, I still have to do normal adult things. I still have to shower. I still have to show up to appointments on time. I even have to buy groceries and return my library books. Seriously, the struggle . . .

Don't worry- I realize I am not "Tiffany- Queen of Suffering." I know that I am not the only person who struggles with fatigue. I would guess that my entire crazy, chronic family struggles with fatigue on some level. We all understand what it feels like, and I think we all feel a little helpless about how to control it. Here's what I have learned from my own quest of dealing with fatigue while still trying to adult.

1.   Know your window.

Is there are certain time of day when you're more likely to feel awake than others? If so, that's your window. For me, on a good day I am typically awake and functional from noon until 4 PM. Anything before or after that window requires planning. (Anything strenuous within that window requires planning.) However, if I'm scheduling a doctor's appointment, physical therapy, time with a friend, etc. I aim for my window. Once you figure out your window of awake time (however big or small it may be), it is easier to make plans.

Joe and I don't have "date nights", we have "day trips." If we wait until the normal hours for dating time, I'll be too tired to participate. Instead, we've learned that day trips work better for us. We sleep late and leave around noon. By the time late afternoon/ early evening arrives, we've had our fun, and I'm ready to rest. The last time we had a "date night", I ended up taking a nap at a table in downtown Nashville while Joe listened to music.

That's right, people. I'm the life of the party.

2.   Stock pile rest.

Whoever said that you can't catch up on missed sleep (or get extra rest beforehand to prepare for missed sleep) has clearly never met a person with chronic illness. If I know that I will have a busier day than normal, I'll schedule extra rest time. Sometimes that means that I have to cancel things I would like to do in the days before or after an event, but if that makes me able to do something I really want to do (or need to do) then it's worth it. Besides, if I don't rest before an event, I'll rest *during* the event, and that seems to make people uncomfortable.

Last year, Mother's Day fell days before Joe and I were leaving for Disney World. I knew I couldn't travel home to visit my mom and still get the rest I would need before leaving for Disney. It was one of those frustrating situations that happen with chronic illness where you have to make decisions and compromises and no decision will make you completely happy. In the end, we "rescheduled" Mother's Day. My mom and I celebrated a week early and acted as though it was legitimately Mother's Day. The perk? Restaurants weren't nearly as packed, and there was an awesome selection of bouquets at the store.

3.   Realize you can't always "push through" fatigue.

My body sends me signals that I have pushed too hard for too long. I'll start running a low grade fever. I'll fall asleep sitting up (typically in inconvenient places). My first tendency is always to think, "This will be the time I can outwit my symptoms and avoid a crash." That has never happened. Ever. Our bodies are like the most temperamental of toddlers. Without our rest, we will fall apart, and the meltdown is never pretty.

This past Christmas I overscheduled activities and under scheduled rest- which is basically what everyone does during the holidays. I cooked, cleaned, traveled, shopped, visited, wrapped, and ate until I barely knew what my name was. By the time Christmas came, I was so tired I was hyper-emotional. (Yes, I cried over all the gifts I gave and received. I teared up because the sweet potatoes were delicious. I may have even shed a tear when

Joe threw away a roll I was planning to eat later.) How did it all end? Projectile vomiting all through Christmas night followed by two weeks of a fever and worsened symptoms. A fatigue meltdown isn't always avoidable. The holidays are difficult and exhausting for everyone. However, I wish I had advocated for myself better. I wish I had declined an invitation or purchased food instead of cooking it. There were opportunities to make the holidays easier on me, and I chose not to take them- and paid dearly for those decisions.

We live in a society that applauds "pushing through" more than it appreciates self-awareness and self-care. I understand that. I understand what our culture wants me to be- but I just CAN'T DO IT. I'm not ashamed by that, though. It is more valuable for me (and those in my life) if I accept my limitations and make the most of the hours I can be productive. The hours that I have to use to recover or rest for the next event are nothing to be ashamed of- they're a necessary part of living my life in spite of my illness.

4.   Napping doesn't actually fix the problem.

I make this mistake a lot. I'm tired; I want to nap. I naively believe that a nap is going to fix the issue of being tired somehow. It doesn't. That's how chronic fatigue works. No amount of sleep is going to fix this situation. It's a permanent state of being. My best advice is to nap when you need it and save your energy for things that really matter. I may spend the majority of my day napping before I attend my 8 year old nephew's basketball game. It's not that I think napping is going to make me less tired, but it will keep me from expending energy that I would rather spend watching my sweet nephew play a game he enjoys. In my experience, a nap is more of a low energy trade-off to pass the time.

5.   Operate in Energy Saving Mode.

This isn't *always* possible. Some activities require that you be fully functional, but I've learned there are a few shortcuts. (For example, if I shower the night before an event, my hair has all night to dry, and I don't have to waste precious energy blow drying my hair.) I realize that you've probably been told your entire life to avoid shortcuts, but it's time to be practical. If getting ready to go out is going to make you too tired to actually go out, find a short cut! Wear a hat; put on dark sunglasses; throw a scarf over your grungiest sweatshirt to make it cuter. Do what you have to do in order to enjoy yourself.

I cook for my husband and I (as well as my husband's parents) a few days a week. I'm glad to contribute to my family by doing something I enjoy (and I think I'm pretty good at it- I mean, I've not killed anyone yet, and I don't think my current health status is a reflection of my cooking skills . . .). However, if I'm being honest, there are so many days that I am tempted to just order a pizza. The problem isn't that I dislike cooking; the problem is that cooking requires so much more energy than I actually have. Fortunately, I've found ways to cook in energy saving mode. For example, did you know that you can buy onions, potatoes, and peppers pre-chopped? Yeah, that's a real thing. Yes, it's more expensive, but it's completely worth it. Also, you can put almost anything into a slow cooker, and it comes out edible hours later. Clearly, my cooking is far from gourmet, but we haven't starved yet. I could expend more energy to cook a really impressive meal, but then I would never get anything else accomplished.

When you operate in energy save mode, there are a lot of trade-offs. Some days I have to skip a shower if I'm going to be able to go to the grocery store. (I'm convinced God created dry shampoo with me in mind.) Other days I have to skip cooking dinner if I'm going to be able to attend a function with my husband that evening. I'm constantly missing one thing I want to do in order to do something else I want to do more, and I've learned to live with that. If not, I would do everything for a couple days, and then spend a couple weeks recovering. That's definitely not worth it.

6.   Communicate.

At least eighty percent of my problems in life could be solved with better communication. I'm embarrassed that I can't hold it together as well as my peers, so I try to hide it. No one is asking me to hide the fact that I have limitations beyond those of my same aged friends, but I feel like everyone is tired of hearing about it. I *know* I'm tired of telling them about it. However, my friends, family, and spouse deserve to know if my window is limited that day. It's unfair of me to plan 4 hours of activities with someone when I know I only have 2 hours of energy. I'll be lifeless for the last 2 hours; my friend will feel guilty, and it will all be my fault.

Think of it this way, expecting someone else to notice when you're getting too tired to function is like expecting someone else to know when you need to use the restroom. You would never let someone make restroom decisions for you, because you know that no one knows your body and how it feels. Concerning fatigue, no one can possibly understand how you're feeling either. As your need increases, they won't know about it, and this will end in a potentially embarrassing and messy situation- much like our hypothetical bathroom example.

At this point, I have accepted my fatigue as a vital part of who I am. It owns me. My decisions are all made through a filter of "How tired am I right now?" It's a complicated way to live life, and I certainly don't recommend it for the faint of heart, but I can't really change it. All I can do is find ways to make my limitations as tolerable as possible. It's all any of our crazy, chronic family can do. In the meantime, I'm thinking of passing around applications for friends who will spend time with me by napping most of the day with an occasional low energy adventure within my window.

That's not too much to ask, is it?

Chronic Pain

Physicians describe chronic pain as pain that lasts longer than six months (webmd.com). Many definitions will go on to say the pain can be localized or general and can vary from mild to excruciating. I realize that definition is accurate, but it falls short of explaining how I really feel. Everything hurts. If I were to sit here and take an inventory of my body, I would realize I have a painful spot (or spots) on each extremity and, honestly, even my scalp hurts. There are many reasons why members of the chronic illness community are in pain. For example, I have Ehlers Danlos Sydrome-which causes my ligaments to hold my joints too loosely- and my joints dislocate. I have at least one joint dislocation daily, and it isn't unusual to have several in a day. Other members of our community experience nerve pain- which as I understand it is miserable. Some of our friends experience pain from inflammation in their joints or organs. There are probably a hundred more reasons that cause pain to be an issue for the chronically ill. Regardless of the reason, most of those in our crazy, chronic family live in chronic pain.

Pain isn't a popular conversation. As a matter of fact, people want to hear about my pain about as much as they want to hear their racist uncle's political opinions. I don't fully understand why pain is such a taboo topic, but I know that it's something I'm nervous to mention. I rarely mention my pain to my doctor, because I feel like chronic pain somehow discredits me as a patient with legitimate health concerns. I feel like the second I bring up pain control I will be dismissed as a medication seeker.

I realize we live in the age of addiction. I also understand that there are people in the world who abuse narcotic pain medication. I'll be honest; that makes me angry. Don't get me wrong; I understand that addiction is a disease, and I have compassion for those who battle with addiction. Having said that, it stinks that I can't be honest with my doctor without feeling like I am being labeled an addict- even though I have never given him reason to doubt the legitimacy of my ailments.

At this point, I have made the decision not to take narcotic pain medicine to manage my daily pain. Of course, if I have acute pain from an injury, surgery, etc that is a different situation entirely. Right now, my fear of addiction is greater than my physical pain. I won't promise you that will always be the case. I have friends who use narcotic pain medicine to

31

handle their chronic pain. They do so responsibly and under a doctor's instruction and care. I hold absolutely no judgment for their decision, and I applaud their recognition of their how much their physical suffering influenced their lives. It's a decision not to be made on a whim, and it's a decision many of us will make multiple times over the course of our illness.

Pain affects everything.

Pain affects my memory. The other day I was making scrambled eggs. I put the eggs in a pan and placed the pan on the burner. Somewhere in the process of this seemingly mundane task, my neck started hurting so badly I was seeing stars. I stepped away from the stove to look for an ice pack, heating pad, shot of bourbon (joking!), anything to relieve my pain. In my frantic wandering for relief, I forgot about my eggs. A couple minutes later I noticed a funky smell- yep, my eggs! Fortunately, I didn't burn the house down. (My standards for a successful day aren't really that high anymore.) The truth of the matter is that some days my brain is so busy trying to comprehend the amount of pain I'm feeling that it fails to do much else.

Pain affects fun. Joe and I live for fun adventures. We spend our entire year saving and planning for our summer vacation to Disney World. I love

Disney World, and my heart flutters with excitement (I hope that's why it's fluttering anyway) just thinking about it. However, my memories of last year's trip are clouded by memories of pain. Don't get me wrong; I had an incredible time. However, even using my wheelchair, my neck throbs from holding my head upright. My shoulders dislocate if I forget and try to propel myself in the wheelchair. My knees ache from bending. Joe, my own personal Hodor (Game of Thrones reference, anyone?), cannot possibly push my wheel chair smoothly enough to save me from pain, and that's a constant frustration for both of us. No matter how much fun we have, the reality of my chronic pain is still there.

Pain affects plans.

Pain is rude. It never calls ahead to let you know it's coming; it just shows up in all its obnoxious glory. It's *very* rare that I cancel plans because of pain. If I did, it would be a slippery slope to total isolation. However, on the rare occasion I'm in too much pain to function one day, I can't plan for it. I have no clue when I go to bed at night if the next day will be excruciating- or a normal day with just intense pain.

Even if I don't cancel due to pain, I'm not exactly the life of the party when I'm trying to keep my hips in socket. That's the problem. Pain isn't something you can just ignore. Pain demands to be felt. Pain acts like a toddler yelling for your attention; it keeps getting louder/more intense as you ignore it. Eventually, it will prove impossible to ignore. At that point, pain has ruined your plans- even if you showed up and tried to do everything.

A couple years ago I accompanied my nephew (then 7) to an interactive museum where he used a wand to cast spells and unlock different rooms. It was the type of place that should make my Harry Potter loving heart want to sing and dance. My nephew was so pumped to cast his spells and explore the castle. I wanted to be excited; I was aware that the whole experience was pretty awesome. However, I was recovering from a dislocated hip and torn hip labrum. What do I remember? Limping behind him and looking for a water fountain to take more ibuprofen. It happens. I showed up and tried to keep our plans, but it certainly didn't go as planned.

Pain affects relationships.

It's tough to have a healthy relationship with a person when you're constantly distracted by trying to hold yourself together. Joe is so used to me falling apart that he's been known to say things like, "Get that knee back in so we can go." Yep, friends, that's the kind of empathy you can expect from marriage. It's fine, really. It's ridiculous to expect him to weep and mourn over every injury. He would spend his whole day bemoaning my illness, and my life requires that I do plenty of that nonsense.

Please don't think Joe is the only insensitive person in our marriage. Joe, for whatever reason, cannot function when he has a headache. To be honest, I have absolutely no clue if he gets especially ill with a headache or if he's an enormous headache diva. (For the sake of fairness, he handles other types of pain better. He's a champ with pulled muscles. I really think he would probably handle a broken leg better than he handles a headache.) All I know is when has a headache, he goes to bed. He literally closes the curtains, puts on his pajamas, and gets in bed. That baffles me. I can't remember a day without a headache in the past five years. My empathy is broken, and it affects how I treat the person I love most in this world.

Pain affects my personality.

Before my symptoms became unavoidable, I was a middle/ high school teacher. If you've ever spent much time around a child between the ages of 12-18, you know they require an enormous amount of patience. I used to be that person. I'm not anymore. Not only do I not teach anymore, I don't have that patience level either. I try to be that person. I hope and pray that I am a kind and graceful person, but I am aware that a lot of who I am is marred by the pain I endure daily.

I'm more emotional now than I've ever been in my life. Sometimes the most ridiculous things will send me into tears. It's not necessarily that I've suddenly become more easily upset than before, but I already feel like I live on the verge of tears. It doesn't take much to push me over the ledge.

See what I mean? Pain affects *everything*.

It wouldn't be fair of me to tell you all the ways pain makes my life difficult and then not give any advice for handling it. I promised you a crazy, chronic guide to dealing with symptoms, right?

1.   Don't compare suffering.

I learn this lesson a little more each day. Pain is pain, and it all hurts. If you've pulled a muscle and someone else broke their leg, yes, their pain is probably greater than yours. However, that doesn't make your pain any less. You still have to deal with your own pain. You're not wrong or inconsiderate for recognizing your own pain. I hear people say a lot that 'it can always be worse.' Yes, it probably can, but if it's already bad it's okay to acknowledge that.

Also, give your non-chronic pain friends (or spouse, in my case) a break. Just because their pain seems insignificant compared to the magnitude of pain you endure, that doesn't mean it doesn't hurt. Just because someone else's pain is less than yours that doesn't mean it isn't traumatic for them. Try to resist the urge to compare what someone else is going through to what you've endured.

2.   Find a doctor you can talk to honestly.

God bless the doctors that don't act like I'm crazy when I mention the pain I feel. There's a therapeutic value in having a doctor who acts like he or she believes me. One sympathetic nod and I'm over the moon! (The first doctor who says something along the lines of "I'm so sorry you're dealing with that" is my date to Christmas dinner!) Trust me, even if you're like me and don't feel ready to start trying pharmaceutical pain relief measures, you still need

37

someone who tries to understand your struggle. You deserve to have a doctor that you don't feel like you're hiding the truth from. When and if the day comes that you need more aggressive pain management, your history will be documented.

Furthermore, there is no shame in seeing a pain management specialist. Do your research beforehand to ensure the doctor you are seeing is prepared to handle your specific disorder. Personally, I think it's brave to admit you need help in order to live your life more fully. If you need someone to help you deal with the pain you feel, speak up and advocate for yourself. A pain management specialist may be able to offer helpful treatment.

### 3.	Comfort matters more than style.

Years ago I had the most fabulous collection of shoes. I had high heels in virtually every color, sandals with bling, and wedges that made me look six inches taller. Now, if I wear shoes that are the least bit uncomfortable, I'll be icing my knees and ankles for days afterward. I've accepted that I'll be wearing flat shoes forever (sigh . . .). For chronic pain sufferers, we have enough struggles just to function. It's ridiculous to add to the struggle with clothes, shoes, makeup, or whatever causes you more discomfort.

4.   Notice your pain patterns.

Let me be clear, your pain is not your fault. I'm not suggesting that you should find the pattern, so you can stop doing the things that cause you pain. It's not that simple; I know that. However, there are certain patterns I've noticed, and I try to avoid triggers if I can. For example, I always have more pain if I sit upright for a long time. I've learned to change positions frequently and lie down on occasion to minimize the pain flair (Super convenient in public, right?). I've also noticed that I feel worse when the atmospheric pressure is low. If I know low pressure is coming into the area, I'll try to get errands and appointments done beforehand. That doesn't help me avoid the pain, but it at least keeps me from having to deal with pain while completing a list of errands.

5.   Don't be embarrassed by your pain.

Even well-meaning people will say insensitive things in regard to the pain you feel. I'm 31, and I occasionally hear, "Just wait until you're older. You don't know what pain is yet." Maybe that's true, but I have my doubts. Regardless, none of us asked for this. I'm not ashamed of my pain, and you don't have to be ashamed of yours. It's not something I discuss a lot, because it would make for boring conversation. However, I also don't have to hide it as though it's a really embarrassing family member. No. It's a part of me. I don't want it, but I'm stuck with it. If you're in too much pain to do something you have scheduled, there's no need for guilt or shame. You're doing the best you can to function on a daily basis. If you swing and miss today, you'll get it tomorrow or the next day. I promise.

There's no shame in however you choose to treat your pain either. Of course, I believe a medical professional should handle all pain management, but if you and your doctor decide you need to treat your pain aggressively- do it. There is nothing wrong with taking a narcotic pain medicine if your doctor recommends it.

There is nothing wrong with trying an alternative or holistic treatment if that is what your medical team thinks you need. It's time that we let go of our notions of how we're supposed to handle pain, because life doesn't exactly prepare us for these moments. Find a doctor you trust; do what is best for you, and don't worry about anyone else's opinion of your treatment.

The problem of pain is difficult. Every person feels pain in one way or the other, so people who live outside our world of chronic pain tend to oversimplify what we're handling. The truth is that chronic pain is a daily struggle that affects every part of our lives and relationships. There are no easy answers on how to manage this. It's a day to day and person to person decision, and as long as you're doing your best, there is no wrong way to handle it.

Bodily Fluids, Functions, and General Funk

This may be the chapter that makes my mother cringe- and wonder how she failed to raise a lady. If so, I get it. What kind of weirdo talks about *all* their bodily functions in print? Yeah, me. On the other hand, some of you may have turned to this chapter first- if that's you, let's be besties. Please? I love a person who can appreciate a friendly discussion on urine.

Okay, here's the truth. If you live with a chronic illness, more than likely some kind of general bodily funkiness is a part of your daily life. One day it's constipation; the next day the problem is a lovely rash. It's always something. For me, it's become such a part of my life that if you're in my inner circle of friends, we *are* going to discuss bodily fluids/functions. Is that gross? Heck, yeah. Is it my reality? Yeah, I'm afraid so.

Urine Trouble (You're in trouble . . . See what I did there?)

My bladder issues are something I've never discussed openly. I'm not ashamed by my struggle; it's not like I have a choice in whether this happens. It just makes everyone else uncomfortable, so I try to spare them details. I realize how bizarre it is that the first time I chose to share

this story is in a book, but I have a flair for the dramatic like that.

Roughly a year into my chronic illness journey- when I was still

undiagnosed- I was driving home from work, and I started peeing. It was

the oddest experience. I was sitting at a red light waiting to turn left (I

have such strange and specific memories of this moment), and I started

peeing on myself! I had a 35 minute drive through the country with no gas

stations for quick restroom stops (Although, really, what was the point

now?), so I just drove home in my wet jeans feeling like an idiot. When I

got home, I stood in the bathroom in disbelief, and I remember praying,

"God, please don't let this become a *thing*" as I took my wet clothes to

the washer.

Yeah, it definitely became a *thing*- an unavoidable, undeniable thing. I hid

the whole mess (quite literally) from my husband for a while, because I

was so embarrassed. Few things can make you feel as insecure as losing

control of a basic bodily function that you've been in control of for a

while. I felt so infantile as I would make mad dashes to the restroom to try

to hide yet another sprung leak. Each new "urinary surprise" resulted in a

new meltdown. Once, in a moment of frustration and rage I threw my wet underwear at the washer, missed the washer completely, and they (along with the cleaning products on the shelf above the washing machine) landed behind the machine. We left that apartment years ago, and I probably owe an apology to the current residents for the urine soaked panties that live behind the washer. (I *could* have asked Joe to make the washing machine so I could get them out, but that would have required telling him what was going on.)

Eventually, I had to tell Joe what was happening. As my problem escalated, it became impossible to hide leak guards, frantic runs to the bathroom (and I am *not* a pretty sight when I run anywhere- Yikes!), and my tendency to burst into angry tears at every bathroom visit. Besides, I was haunted by nightmares where Joe and I were about to have, um, intimacy (Yes, I can speak freely about pee but saying "sex" makes me blush for days. Good grief.) and I peed on him. No, that never actually happened, but I was terrified it would. Here's the thing- I told Joe and his reaction was, "Okay, if you need pads or whatever from the store you'll have to text me a picture. I won't know what to get." That probably sounds like an insensitive response, but it's what I needed. If he had held me and let me cry over everything that was happening in my life, I would have probably never stopped crying.

Opening up about my struggle was my first step to getting some semblance of a new kind of normalcy. Once Joe knew about my "pee problems," he encouraged me to find a doctor to help with the situation. I visited several doctors and tried many new medicines- all without significant improvement. I've had tests to diagnose my problem and procedures to try fixing it. I had a bladder pacemaker implanted months ago with some success.

Here's the thing- my "urine trouble" is still bothersome. It's the one symptom that embarrasses me most. There are still days that I look at myself in the mirror and tell myself that I'm disgusting. It's not true, but this whole situation is a lot to handle. Even though I truly have no control over what my bladder does, I still feel embarrassed by it from time to time. However, after several years of dealing with these issues, I've come to accept it and even joke about it. If Joe and are traveling and he asks if I need to use the restroom, I always tell him I went about 15 minutes ago. When he reminds me that it's been two hours since we stopped, I'll say, "Yes, I'm aware." It's silly, but for me, once I can joke about something, I can accept it and move on.

Poop (Wait, can I use the word "poop" in a book? I have no idea if this is okay!)

While we're discussing the leakage of the lower orifices, let's go ahead and cover movements of the bowel variety. Now, if you're like me (and a lot of my chronic illness friends) there's not a lot to say about poop, because it happens with about as much frequency as a lunar eclipse. Unfortunately for my friends, my movements get about as much press coverage (by me- not local media) as an eclipse too. You've officially moved out of the friend zone and into the bestie zone when I text to let you know my body has called off its moratorium on expelling waste. It's a call for celebration.

I'm trying to spare you unnecessary detail, but a portion of my health status from day to day depends on my digestion. New foods are terrifying, because I have no clue how my body will respond from a digestive perspective. There's a chance I could spend the rest of the day in the restroom- or there's a chance my next restroom trip will be two weeks away. So, even though this all a little gross to mention, it's a legitimate concern in our everyday lives that had to be discussed.

Vomit

My initiation to the life of the chronically ill came in the form of a night of vomit. My story started there, and I have since "tossed my cookies" in every possible place. I've thrown up in every restaurant restroom in our small town, at my old job, at Joe's office, at church, every store in town, and at virtually every gas station along the I-75 stretch from Kentucky through Tennessee. It's annoying, but I'm always prepared. I keep nausea medication, mints, wet wipes, make up, and a toothbrush with me at almost all times. I've even become very organized about the way I vomit (typically). I can step away from the table, walk to the restroom, lose my lunch, and return to the table in under ten minutes. I'm efficiently ill at least.

I've tried everything to handle the situation. I ate gluten free for six months- MORE vomit than before. (Most of my safe, bland foods contain gluten. Without them, I was lost.) I've had a liquid diet of smoothies and Gatorade- no significant relief. I don't *always* throw up. I, instead, go in strange cycles of the "upchuck life" and then blessed weeks when it doesn't happen. While I have some definite food aversions that make my stomach funky (Pancakes, why must you always make me so very sick?), I realize there's a little more to it now. If I'm excessively tired, I vomit. If I'm dealing with too much stress, I vomit. If I get too warm, I vomit. Are you seeing a pattern? Basically, I'm a bit like an inking sea creature- except with vomit. If my body feels threatened in any way, it projectile vomits in self-defense. My stomach has obvious ninja-like skills.

General Funk

What the heck is "general funk"? Well, it's the catchall section for all the other random body grossness that happens to us. At some point, my body began throwing a wild, drunken party and forgot to invite me. The party serves headaches and nausea and decorates with colorful rashes and bruises. These lovely decorations (and other various "party favors") are the general funk.

Rashes

At some point almost every day, I'll notice hives, blotches, or some other strange skin deformity. It's just decoration; it never means anything significant. My body just occasionally erupts into odd blotches. Again, it seems to all coincide with exhaustion, but that's clearly unavoidable. I'm learning not to even react to it anymore. I used to take pictures to ask my doctor about it, but by now I've just accepted my blotchiness as part of the party. Yes, there are the occasional moments of others asking, "Ew!

What's that?!?" My favorite response is, "Oh nothing. Just glad to see you." It makes all of us equally uncomfortable.

Sounds

The wild, drunken party raging inside my body is noisy- always. Let's imagine for a moment that I am going to go from sitting to standing. First, my lower back will pop; then my toe will crack as I try to steady my feet before standing. Finally, my knees and hips will join the party with grinding sounds of their own. I'm a human Rice Krispies commercial (Snap! Crackle! Pop!). It's ridiculous. Occasionally, I get comments from super helpful people telling me I'm too young for my joints to be so noisy. Yeah, thanks. I'm fully aware.

On the occasion that I don't have to move, then my bones/ joints are quiet (unless I'm sitting up- then my neck will pop every time I turn my head). That's when my stomach decides to wage war with itself. For a person with ridiculously slow digestion, somehow when I get in public the whole process decides to announce itself. My stomach rumbles; my throat gurgles, and if I'm not careful a very unladylike belch will escape (Oh, good grief, let's hope that's all that escapes!). I'm basically no longer meant for human interaction.

This is the part where I'm supposed to give you advice on how to handle all this bodily funk that's happening to you, but to be honest, I'm still figuring it out. It sort of happens on a case by case basis too. Some days the situation can be handled by an "Oh, excuse me!" Other days, when you've just vomited on a total stranger's shoes, well, I don't even know what to tell you. Smile? Shrug? Burst into tears? There's not a great option. Here's what I have learned though.

1.   **Don't do anything new on a day when you can't afford a bodily rebellion.** If it's your wedding day, if you have the biggest interview of your life, or if you're headed on a first date- don't decide that's the day you want to try something new. Perhaps your digestive system will love calamari, but if it doesn't, you don't want to find out at a crucial time. Perhaps a spin class will be your new favorite thing, but if it isn't, you don't want to pay the price when everything is on the line.

2.   **It's not nearly as obvious as you think.** I have to remind myself on a daily basis that the world doesn't actually revolve around me. It doesn't revolve around you either. (I know, I was crushed by that news too!) That's good news, though. It means

that everyone else isn't noticing your bodily funk nearly as much as you are. Even though you feel like everyone in your office is scandalized by your frequent mad dashes to restroom, they've probably never noticed. Even if you're convinced your breath reeks of vomit (or your pants reek of urine), more than likely, no one knows but you. Trust me- everyone else is so wrapped up in their own hot mess they're probably ignoring yours.

3.   **If something happens and an orifice leaks (in public!), give yourself a break.** I can't say this enough. You can't hold it together all the time. There will probably be a day in your crazy, chronic life when you open your mouth to speak and vomit shoots out. There could be a day when you lose control over lower bodily functions. It happens. You aren't gross or disgusting. Your illness is a jerk, and you're a warrior for fighting it daily. Clean yourself up; binge watch something ridiculous; eat some comfort food. Just don't convince yourself that you're ready to give up- you're way too strong for that.

Crazy, Chronic Survival Guide for Doctor's Appointments

An unfortunate part of every chronic illness life is doctor's appointments. Don't get me wrong; I have some incredible doctors. If we could meet for coffee and discuss the weather or sports (or anything other than how incredibly jacked up my body is), I would genuinely enjoy their company. However, appointments with doctors just aren't fun. First of all, most of my doctors are specialists- which means I only see them a couple times a year. When my appointment time finally rolls around, I have roughly one million questions to ask, and my doctor has approximately 15 minutes to answer all of them. As a result, I often leave feeling disappointed.

This isn't really anyone's fault. I can't blame my doctor for being in high demand. However, it isn't really my fault that I only see him/her every six months or so and, thus, have a lot of questions and high expectations. This survival guide is filled with the things I do to get the most out of appointments while avoiding frustration.

Make a list and check it twice!

I'm not implying that your doctor is like Santa Claus, but he/she does have the power to help you if you work together. Before you go make a list of questions you need to ask. Then, read through the list and remove things that aren't as important or don't apply to the doctor's specialty. For example, if you're seeing your neurologist and you have a weird rash on your foot- probably not worth putting on the list. I realize that may seem obvious, but there are times when I feel like I have to tell the doctor *everything* that's going on, and sadly, for those of us with complex conditions, that's probably not possible in a short time slot.

Also, it's okay if you don't make it all the way through your list. Tell your doctor that you have several things to discuss. If he/she knows they can't discuss that many things, they'll let you know. Then you can choose what is most important to your health at this point. If discussing everything requires a second appointment, that's okay.

Take advantage of patient portals.

One of my favorite innovations in patient care is the advent of the patient portal. Portals allow you to see lab results, view upcoming appointments, and communicate with your doctor. If you have a health issue that comes up and your appointment is still months away, message your doctor. Even if your doctor can't see you to address the concern, the issue will be documented. Sometimes doctors will move your appointment time, so that you can be seen sooner. Regardless, you're doing your best to keep your doctor in the medical loop with you. (Warning- Try to minimize your correspondence via portal. While it's great to let your doctor know what's going on; you don't want to become the patient that floods their inbox daily- unless it's absolutely necessary.)

Keep your expectations in check.

If you've been dealing with an issue for the past 5 months, it's unlikely your doctor will figure it out in 15 minutes. Be realistic. Ask for help but understand that help might not be immediate. If there is something that absolutely needs to be addressed *right now*, let your doctor know that is your biggest concern currently. More than likely it will still take some tests to get an accurate diagnosis and treatment, but at least the ball is rolling.

Remember, you're the consumer.

If you have a concern that you feel your doctors are not addressing, it's perfectly acceptable to find a new doctor that better understands your needs. I'm not a fan of "doctor shopping," and I certainly try to stick with a doctor as long as possible. However, if a doctor is not giving you adequate care, it's time to find a new one. Doctors are human, and they make mistakes. There is, however, a certain standard of care that you should expect. If you don't feel that your doctor is actively trying to better your quality of life, find a new one.

Ultimately, we, as patients, need doctors as part of our care team. There are things we can do to be the best possible patient, and I truly hope that helps us to have the best care possible.

Becoming a "Professional Sick Person

October 26 is my sick-iversary. Technically October 26 isn't the day I became sick, but it was the day that I (or more specifically my doctor) realized that I was too sick to work. I had come to a place where I could no longer do my job as well as I wanted. I was too tired to drive to work. I was too tired and sick to teach when I got there. And, I was too tired and sick to do all the extra parts of my job (attending sporting events, school dances, choir concerts, etc) that I had always enjoyed doing. The realization was hard to arrive at, because I *loved* my job. You see, I was a middle/ high school Spanish teacher, and I am one of those weird people that actually enjoys teenagers. (That's not a plea for any of you to send your children to me, though! I especially love teenagers for 6-7 hours a day when I know I can send them home afterward and let their parents deal with them!) I didn't want to leave. I would have continued to teach forever (and eventually been buried on the football field holding my dry erase markers . . .), but there were a few things that let me know that I *couldn't* do it any longer.

When you work in the education world, you spend a lot of time trying to make everything fair for everyone. You're constantly asking yourself, "Did I call on as many boys as girls to answer questions? Did the last test give students of all learning styles an opportunity to be successful? Do underprivileged students have an equal opportunity for success in my classroom?" My former life revolved around fairness. However, I came to a point where I realized that continuing in the classroom was unfair to everyone involved. At some point, it became selfish to continue working when there were other options that were far more fair and beneficial to everyone involved.

I wasn't being fair to myself.

I taught for over a year while I was very sick. I don't mean that I was really tired (which I was) or I had a headache (which I did). I mean, I was really, really sick. My students were totally used to the fact that I had to step out of class to vomit quite often. My mind would go blank, and I would drop whatever I was holding. Many evenings I had no memory of what had happened during the day when I returned home. In the evening I would go straight to bed, and I was rarely able to leave my bed during the weekend. It was a miserable existence.

The school where I worked was about forty minutes from my house, and I came to a point where I could no longer safely drive there. Joe drove me for a while . . . until I found out the other teachers thought he was driving me because I had a secret DUI! (Good grief.) Fortunately, a few colleagues that also commuted had pity on me (and realized I wasn't a raging alcoholic) and invited me to carpool with them. I was the lamest carpool member ever. I couldn't drive, because I couldn't stay awake (or remember where I was going). I contributed to gas funds every week, but I always felt guilty that we never used my car for the journey. Also, I *always* fell asleep riding to and from work. I hoped that no one noticed (or that they thought it was part of my supposed drinking problem), but I'm fairly confident they couldn't help but notice the semi-conscious carpool member in the back seat leaving drool stains on their leather interior. I was ashamed of the person I had become, but I felt like there was truly nothing I could do about it.

I became self-conscious about hiding how much I was struggling. I taught in a middle and high school, and the schools were separated by a parking lot. I had a five minute break between the end of my middle school classes and the beginning of the high school class time. I had five minutes to walk my middle school students to the library (in a straight and orderly line, because that's how it's done in the middle school world), walk across a parking lot, go up a flight of stairs, and get into my classroom. I couldn't do it. I just couldn't do it. I would black out walking across the parking lot. My knees and hips would hurt so badly by the time I got to the high school that my eyes would be watering. By the time I got to the top of the stairs and started down the hallway to my classroom, I was gasping for breath, nauseous, and at least five minutes late. The high school principal sent several e-mails telling me I needed to get to my class earlier (because high school students can cause some serious mayhem when left to their own devices for five minutes), but I could not get there any faster. In a "normal" situation, I could have just told the principal I was physically incapable of getting there in the amount of time allotted, but I was too ashamed.

I wasn't being fair to my husband.

You know by now that my first major illness meltdown was on my honeymoon, and after that meltdown I've never really been the same. So my time of working while sick was during the first year and a few months of my marriage. As a result, the months when we should have been enjoying each other, making plans for our collective future, and having our first arguments, I

58

was asleep. I would come in from work, and Joe would have dinner prepared.

Let me interject here, that Joe is *not* a cook. He knew, though, that if he waited for me to fix something it would never happen. Essentially we were living off pizza rolls and frozen lasagna, but without those options I probably would not have eaten at all. One night he was very proud of himself for successfully making sloppy joes and macaroni and cheese. An hour after we ate, I was heaving it up in the bathroom while Joe apologized from the hallway for killing me with his cooking. We would eat whatever was in the bounds of his limited (but much appreciated) cooking repertoire, and I would fall asleep eating. I would sleep on the couch until time to move to the bed. Joe was taking care of the cooking, most of the cleaning, packing my lunch, starting my car, and doing everything while I slept. He even went so far as to set up a playlist of my favorite songs to get me pumped up before I left for work. (I have to admit, sick or not, I felt pretty dang cool leaving home to my very own exit music.)

Weekends became more and more difficult. Joe and I are football season ticket holders at the University of Tennessee. I knew when I married Joe that he's a Vols Superfan, and my life would always include attending games in the fall. But it was getting harder and harder to hold up my end of that deal. I was so tired on weekends that I couldn't get out of bed- let alone attend a football game. One weekend I tried to accompany Joe to a game (The university is three hours from the town where we live, so attending a game requires a hotel stay.). I was so sick by half time that we had to leave and watch the second half from our hotel room. Another weekend I was too tired to attend a football game at the university where Joe works, so he went to it alone- his department was hosting a tailgate part for students and other guests. He ended up leaving early, because I called him from the emergency room a couple hours later. (I went in for routine labs, and my heart rate was in the 140s so they kept me for observation.) I wasn't me anymore. I was trying so hard, but I was truly ruining every plan we made. Joe is a trooper, and he married me for better/worse, sickness/health, etc., but he deserved better.

I wasn't being fair to my students.

Do you remember those awful teachers from growing up that sat behind their desks and never moved? The most they ever did was yell at a kid for talking then go back to just sitting there supervising. Yeah, I remember those too, and I vowed to myself when I began teaching that I would never become the teacher that was so tired of teaching that I quit doing my job, but I kept coming to work. But as my health declined, I was becoming more and more like the type of teacher I swore I would never be. I don't think I yelled at students or stopped actually teaching, but I was definitely lifeless. I went

60

from being the type of teacher that taught students silly songs and dances to remember new concepts to being the kind of teacher that hoped she had enough worksheets planned to keep students from planning a mutiny.

For the first time in my professional life, I was getting less than perfect evaluations. The administrators were saying things like, "The students really enjoy her class . . . but wish she was here more." I had never been a teacher that used my sick days- even when I should have! Years before all this, I was actually standing in front of my class teaching when I received a phone call telling me I had tested positive for swine flu. (In my defense, I thought I was having an asthma flare and couldn't possibly be contagious.) I was mortified that my superiors possibly thought I had a poor work ethic. Even though I always communicated with my colleagues if I had a doctor's appointment that would cause me to miss work, I still felt the shame associated with my absences.

Before the days of illness, I was the kind of teacher that went to student sporting events, academic team matches, choir and band concerts, plays . . . I sponsored snowball dances and prom and free tutoring sessions in my classroom. I even missed my students during long weekends. I really believe I was created to teach. But, when you're struggling to stay conscious and vomiting between class periods, you lose some of your drive. As I became sicker and sicker, I became less and less of the teacher I wanted to be. The students I had during those last few horrible months deserved the best of me, and that was a part of me that was no longer available.

I had to stop working, and I lost so much of myself when I did. I identified myself as a teacher, because that's what I always wanted to be. I had spent years of my life (and a good chunk of my parents' savings) training to make that dream a reality. I value my role as a wife, as a daughter, as a sister, and as a friend, but I still felt I was a teacher primarily. If someone asked me who I was or what did, I proudly stated, "I teach." I didn't say I cook, I clean, I write, or I care for my family and friends. I was primarily a teacher, and every other classification lined up somewhere behind that title. Honestly, even though I have not taught in a few years now, I'm still trying to figure out how to explain who I am. I catch myself saying, "I used to be a teacher" or "I'm a teacher, but I'm on a break because of my health." I know that I am more than a 'has been' teacher, but I'm still trying to figure it out. Joe still calls me a teacher and insists that I will always be an educator in some capacity (even if the only education I'm imparting is laundry instruction for him). I'm not sure how comfortable I am with the title any more, though.

I still mourn the person I was, but I am also proud of the person I am becoming. I was afraid that I would never be *me* again after I left work. I joke that I am a "professional sick person," and some days I really earn the title. But being a "sick person" doesn't define me the way being a teacher did. I am a wife; I am a daughter; I am a friend. I'm no longer a teacher, and that's okay. I am learning how to be me in spite of the things I miss.

In leaving work, I reclaimed part of my life. I can stay awake to talk to Joe during dinner now, and I can sometimes actually make our dinner. (Thank goodness! No one over the age of twenty can live on a diet of pizza rolls!) I think I'm a bit more pleasant than I was during those awful months of trying to teach while so terribly, chronically ill. I am able to make it to doctor's appointments and treatments without worrying about calling a substitute teacher. I can at least be tired and exhausted at my house where I can nap rather than trying to juggle my fatigue and nausea while teaching Spanish to thirty teenagers. As much as I hate to admit it, even my former students were better off after I left the classroom. I was replaced by instructors who had the energy and enthusiasm I lacked and that my students definitely deserved. This new life isn't always as fulfilling as the one I had before. It is hard to know how to even define success when you're a "professional sick person." Ultimately, though, this life is better than the one I had before; this life is more fair to my husband, my former students, and me.

Things I've learned that might help others-

63

1.   You are more than your career, more than your role in your family, and more than your diagnosis. Never forget that.

2.   You have to make decisions based on what is best for you and your relationships.

3.   Even if something is your absolute passion in life, it's possible to come to a place where you can't do it anymore. Life will go on; it might be painful, but it doesn't end.

4.   If you land your dream job, it will always hold a special place in your heart- even once it's gone. However, that doesn't mean you won't have new dreams and goals afterward. Maybe nothing will ever replace that first love, but you might refocus on a new dream that fulfills you just as much.

5.   Don't look back on what you've lost with sadness; look back and smile at the fun times and positive impact you had while it lasted.

What to do when you can't do anything

Chronic illness essentially means that you spend more time sick than you spend well. That's our lives, and we know how to function in spite of it. There are times, however, when everything is just worse than normal. There are times when you're stuck in bed or on the couch, and there's no hope for productivity in the near future. Maybe you've been "normal people sick" and that set off a flair of your chronic illness. Maybe you've traveled, and you're just absolutely exhausted (more than normal, that is). Whatever the reason, there will be days or even weeks in the chronic illness journey when you can't do anything, and eventually naps will fail to meet their intended purpose.

Learn something new.

If you can't accomplish anything except lying on the couch, put this time to good use and learn something new. Years ago, I was in a symptoms flair at the time I found out my brother and sister in law were having a baby girl. I was so excited for them, but I wasn't well enough to go on an all pink shopping spree for the upcoming little one. So, I started watching

YouTube tutorials about making hair bows. At the time, I didn't have any ribbon, hot glue, or thread. I had no plans of actually making bows for a while, but the videos gave me something to do that felt productive. I bookmarked my favorites. I made lists of what I would need. (Just so you know, the only thing more expensive than buying bows for little girls is making them!) When I started to feel better I had a plan in place.

I'm sure that everyone doesn't want to make bows. I'll be honest; even my interest in bow making has waned over the years. However, everyone has something they would like to do. Maybe you're interested in learning a new language; find YouTube videos to learn more. Peruse your local library's web site, and choose books you would like to check out later. Learn about another culture. Teach yourself about a friend's religion. Figure out how to convert Celsius to Fahrenheit. If there's something you want to learn, it's a great time to do it. Make a plan even if you're not up to the execution.

Have some online fun.

Ew! No, not *that* kind of online fun! What are you? A sixth grade boy?

Shop. Do all the shopping. Amazon is my bestie. I love my husband, but don't make me choose between him and Amazon Prime. I don't buy everything; I'm sure you've noticed that being professionally sick doesn't lend itself to the greatest income. I browse, and I fill my cart. If I ever accidentally hit "buy", I'll have a plethora of weirdness showing up at my door. Once post- surgery and pain medicine, I decided to shop. I have no memory of my shopping experience, but I had packages arriving for days! Joe hid my phone when I was medicated after that experience.

Plan a vacation- or a hypothetical vacation. I spend a lot of time dreaming of all the places I would like to go if I were healthy enough. I don't mean that in a sad "Oh poor Tiffany, she'll never live out her dreams" sort of way. I mean, I'm prepared for the good days, and if I ever find a really great price on a trip- I'm going regardless. I also plan for Joe and I to make our yearly Disney World trip. I enter in different possible arrival and departure dates to see which time is most affordable. I plan dinner reservations and peruse menus. Is it strange that I know what I'm eating every night on vacation at least a month before I go? Yes, it's very weird, but it passes my down time.

Play games. At this point, I'm ashamed by how many levels of Candy Crush I've defeated. No adult should spend that much time mindlessly swiping at their phone's screen, but I do. I have spent countless days staring at my phone playing senseless games. I haven't found a single game that helps me grow or become a better person, so I'm not exactly proud of this addiction. However, sometimes when you feel horrible, it's helpful to have small successes. There are days that my biggest accomplishment is beating a really difficult level on Candy Crush. You know what? I'll take it. Any success beats feeling like a failure.

Social media friends are fantastic. Honestly, it would take an entire book to describe how much the online community has helped me to deal with this crazy, chronic life. Social media is 24/7 365 days of the year. There is always someone around that wants to chat. Sometimes that's exhausting, but other times it comforts me. I can join a forum that appeals to my interest. There are forums for the chronically ill, specific illnesses, hobbies, sports fans- essentially, whatever you want to talk about, someone is there to talk about it.

Adult coloring books were made for me.

And on the eighth day God created the adult coloring book. (For clarity, I mean adult level difficulty- not adult themed coloring books.) I love coloring so much. It's somewhat therapeutic. I love the mindless redundancy of running a marker over a page. On days when I feel useless, I feel like I accomplish something when I finish coloring a detailed picture. I realize that's a lame standard for success, but some days it helps if I finish *anything*.

If you're hands won't cooperate to physically color, there are some great
your
coloring apps available. Colorfy is my favorite. I haven't splurged for the paid features, but there are enough freebies to get me through days when I want to be creative and my fingers won't stay in their sockets.

If you're feeling extra creative (or if you're one of those people who is gifted in artistic endeavors), when you can't get out of bed might be a great time to try a new medium. Maybe you always color with markers, and you would like to try shading pencils instead. This is a fantastic opportunity. Also, if there's something you've always wanted to be able to draw, Google it. While you have your markers/ pencils spread around you, go ahead and learn how to draw a penguin, sloth, or hippo. Seriously, you never know when life might require a hand drawn hippo.

If you can't help yourself, help someone else.

I started saying this early in my diagnosis when I felt especially helpless. I'm confident it isn't a Tiffany original quote, but I have no clue where I heard someone say it. Regardless of who said it first, it's been helpful for me. When I feel absolutely terrible, I can't figure out how to make myself feel better. However, I can normally find someone else that would benefit from encouragement (you know, basically all humans everywhere). Here are a few of things I have tried that helped me get through difficult times.

Send an encouraging e-mail (or snail mail). Look through your Facebook newsfeed for a friend that seems to be struggling and send them a message to let them know you're praying for them and sending warm thoughts. Send a letter to a teacher who inspired you as a student. Ask your pastor for a list of people in your community who are shut- in and send them a card. I promise, you'll feel better when you know you made someone else's day a little brighter.

Text a friend going through a rough time. Even if your friends have scattered since you became ill, it's okay to reach out to them. I get it. I've been really hurt by friends who just weren't there when I needed them. However, just because my friends hurt me, I don't want revenge. (Two wrongs don't make a right, you know?) Let your friend know you are available if they want to binge watch Gilmore Girls at your house. Or, if you're not up to seeing them, just a nice text letting your friend know you're thinking about him/ her goes a long way.

Plan an outing or a meal for a family member- execute later. Sometimes when I'm sick, I'll research festivals, educational activities, and general fun for my nephew and niece. I'll send the link to their parents, or I'll plan to take them eventually. Remember, this awful moment of feeling bad won't last forever. Plan for the future. Construct a dinner menu, and invite a friend to join you in cooking it when you're feeling a little better.

Clip coupons. Of course, clipping coupons is great for personal gain. You can hang out on your couch and figure out ways to get free toilet paper forever, and that's perfectly fine. However, if you know a young parent who is struggling, it would be great to clip "baby stuff" coupons for them. (It might be best to ask them if they want the coupons first though.) Clip coupons for school supplies for friends with school age kids. There are plenty of people who would like to coupon, but don't know where to start.

Mentally walk through your house, and make a list of items you can donate to charity once you're feeling better. I know when I'm lying on the couch, I can normally identify how much extra junk my husband and I have accumulated. (It drives me crazy when I feel bad!) Make a list. If there are non-sick people around, have them gather the items on the list and donate them to a charity of your choice. That table you've been tripping over for months might be the first piece of "real" furniture a single mom has in her apartment. Or that stool that is just in the way, maybe what allows a widow to reach the top shelf in her kitchen now that her husband isn't there to hand her the things she can't reach.

If you can't do *anything*, that's fine too.

Please, don't interpret this chapter to mean you have to spend your sickest days doing something. Sometimes you can't. I understand that. The most important thing you can do when you're extra sick is to take care of yourself.

Spend your days sleeping. I'm always amazed by how many hours I can sleep when I'm extra exhausted. About once a month my body crashes and sleeps the greater part of a 24 hour period. It's not exactly exciting, but I assume that's what my body needs. There's not guilt in sleeping your days away.

Be selfish. I'm serious. When you're stuck on the struggle bus, there's no shame in making it all about you. I'm not suggesting you be rude or unkind. I'm simply suggesting that you turn down invitations that require leaving bed until you're able to fully engage again. Let your family eat sandwiches and Hot Pockets for a couple days. It won't kill them; I promise. Let Netflix babysit your children (or spouse). Take care of yourself first. Eat comfort foods. Snuggle in a blanket. Nurture yourself so you can get back to being the person you normally are as soon as possible.

Ask for help. This is so hard for me. I feel guilty asking someone to go out of his way to do a task I normally do. I understand that isn't easy; I really do. However, it's very important that you communicate your needs. If you can't make it to the grocery store, text a list to your spouse. If you can't mow the yard, ask (and pay) the neighbor kid to do it for you. It's okay to ask for help when you need it. As a matter of fact, it's necessary.

Here's the truth- there is no right or wrong way to handle being ill. None of planned for this life, and we would all prefer if our days were a little

us

Edit jobs?

73

more fun. However, when we feel horrible, there has to be something better to do than Googling symptoms and panicking (other people do that too, right?). I don't claim to know exactly how you should spend your day, because I don't think there is an easy answer. Whatever you do, make sure it is a step toward feeling better physically or mentally. If it's a nap, a hobby, or something to encourage someone else, do whatever helps. And on those days when nothing helps, learn to draw a panda, because that sounds awesome.

Crazy, Chronic Survival Guide to Packing and Road Trips

I'm married to the ultimate extrovert. Joe lives for crowds, and he's the

life of the party. Me? Well, I can act nice in public, but I'm spending my

time yearning for the comfort of my Dora the Explorer pillow and a fleece

blanket. We compromise by having a lot of quiet evenings at home and

then making weekend trips whenever possible. Traveling is so hard for

those of us with chronic illness. I'm never sure how to pack, because I

have no idea what kind of curve ball my body will throw while I'm away.

My pain levels are always nearing a breaking point, and a long ride in the

car may push me over that edge. There are so many possible things that

could go wrong- and that doesn't even account for whatever we're

planning to do once we arrive at our destination.

The good news- I've always survived our trips. Some were a bit more

successful than others. Some trips were riddled with bad decisions, but

my record for general survival is still at 100%. While I'm aware that my

standard for a successful trip is pretty low, (What kind of person considers a successful road trip to be any road trip where they didn't actually die?) I'm still sharing my tips. With a little bit of practice in juggling a chronic illness while being Joe's travel partner, I can honestly say that I typically enjoy our adventures- even if I have to pay the price in exhaustion for a few days afterward.

1. **Plan for the worst and hope for the best.** I have a ridiculous amount of luggage when I travel, and I don't apologize for it. When I travel, I make sure I have every possible thing I might need. That means I pack an extra bag of medicine that I don't typically take but I would need in an emergency. I pack more clothes than I'll actually need, because my body has temperature control issues. Do most people require a sweatshirt in July? Of course, not. But, for me, it's a possibility. I also pack cold packs and heating pads, KT tape, anti-itch cream, a battery operated fan, two turtle doves, and a partridge in a pear tree. Okay, something like that.

2. **Comfort is key.** One time I let Joe talk me into riding 15 hours to Nacogdoches, TX. I have no clue what I

was thinking, and I truly hope I'm smart enough not to make that mistake twice. I survived the 30 hour round trip by turning the backseat of our car into a bed. (Don't worry, Mom. I still wore a seat belt, and I did not lean on the door at any time!) Joe helped me cover the backseat with a fluffy queen sized comforter and throw pillows. It wasn't perfect, but it cut down on a lot of the beating and banging that typically happens during car trips. (If only I could always ride in my cozy car/bed . . .)

I also always pack some extra comfortable clothes for the trip. I don't ever intentionally pack uncomfortable clothes, but I travel with the knowledge that there will probably be a day where I'm in so much pain that I can't stand clothes that fit properly. I've often said one of the best parts of marriage is the endless supply of "boy clothes" I can snag. Normally in my suitcase amidst the sundresses and leggings there's at least one pair of Joe's basketball shorts and an oversized t-shirt. Do I always look fabulous? Nope. Not at all. But sometimes comfortable clothes are the only way I can manage to get out of the hotel room, and Joe and I have learned to accept that.

3.   **Appease your anxiety.** I would love to be able to say that I've reached a point in my illness journey where I no longer constantly think about "What ifs". I've not. I worry when we go out of town about how my body will react and where I can get help if I need it. The best way I've found to combat this is to make a plan. When Joe and I schedule *anything*, we also purchase travel protection. That means we can cancel or reschedule a trip if I get ill beforehand. This keeps us from traveling when I absolutely don't need to even try. Some places (like Disney World and most cruise lines) also include in their travel protection plan coverage in case you become ill while you're on the trip. Typically, I can handle my medical drama alone, but I take great comfort in knowing that if I need a doctor, there's a plan in place. If we're visiting a new place, I will do a quick Google search to find out about the hospitals in the area. More than likely, I

won't need a hospital, but I feel better prepared if I've done my homework before I leave.

4. **Make sure your travel group knows your needs.** I haven't been brave enough to travel without my husband or my mom since my symptoms became severe. But, if you're traveling with people who aren't fully aware of your medical needs, let them know beforehand. If you'll need help propelling your wheelchair, make sure your group knows and is prepared to help push you. If you'll be using crutches or a walker to get around, prepare your group for the reality that you may move more slowly than everyone else. If you're not able to keep up with a packed schedule, tell your group beforehand that it's not personal. Most people are wonderful and flexible, but it's best to let them know what you need and expect.

If you travel with a chronic illness, it will most definitely be more difficult than simply staying at home. However, some of my favorite memories were made from doing difficult things. If I weren't willing to endure a little discomfort, I wouldn't have had my wonderful Disney

World experiences. If I were too scared to ever leave the country, I would have never seen blue Caribbean waters with my family. There are a lot of wonderful experiences in this world, and even though I know it will be difficult, I'm not willing to miss out on any of them I can possibly do.

Accepting Disabled Life

What I'm about to say is ridiculous, but bear with me- I've spent most of my life being hopelessly naive. Before I became disabled, I had a completely unrealistic mental picture of what disability is. I imagined that a person who is disabled from illness lived at home, but that home was a pristine- almost clinical- setting. I imagined the person (always a woman in my mind) wore a high-necked pastel gown and sat in her bed propped by pillows. Her hair was clean, and the sheets and pillows smelled of freshly washed linens. A nurse carried medication and small cups of water to this poor, ill soul. Friends and neighbors gathered around hoping to find some way to help the ailing victim of illness.

What the heck, right? Could I have possibly been more wrong about what the professionally sick life actually is? The outrageous part of all this is I knew people who were disabled by illness before it happened to me. I knew that's not how their lives were, but I still had my mental image. The truth of the "sick life" is that it's messy and lonely. There are days when I can't find the energy to shower or even change out of yesterday's pajamas. I wash the sheets when I feel capable of walking up and down the stairs to the laundry room (which means sometimes they sit in the dryer a week before I get the energy to bring them upstairs). Friends and neighbors are typically unaware of my illness- or at least how much it affects me. They're certainly not standing around offering to help. It's not unusual for weeks to pass, and I haven't spoken to anyone besides my mom and my husband. (Thank goodness they're good conversationalists.)

I'm not complaining that disabled life is different than I pictured it. I think the fictitious disabled life I had pictured would get old just as quickly as real disabled life has. Regardless, this life is *not* what I signed up for! I never planned on life turning out this way. I spent years in college training to be a teacher. Heck, I'm still paying student loans. I passed certification tests and went through grueling interviews. I did a lot of work in order to have the job I wanted, and I was blindsided by the sick life. I wasn't prepared for this outcome at all.

It's all so hard to accept. I identified myself as a teacher before anything else, and I will more than likely never teach again. There's a part of me that feels like if I'm not the person I envisioned being, then I have no clue who I actually am. I've been in a cycle of grief over losing myself ever since I first felt my life slipping away because of illness. Some days I think I have finished the cycle and moved past my losses; other days I'm angry and sad all over again. Regardless of how I feel on any day, this is my life now, and I have no choice but to accept it. Railing against it is too exhausting.

For me, the first step to accepting disabled life was to realize I still have a job- even if I don't like it. It's *not* that I don't have a job anymore. It's just that my new job really sucks. I'm professionally sick. I actually receive a check, because I have been deemed too ill to adult. My health has become my new job, and I easily spend eight hours a day working on it.

My job is my health. My health is a delicate balance, and I spend time every day trying to protect that balance. I take medication, go for treatments, schedule and attend doctor's appointments, and even try to maintain an exercise routine. None of that is fun, and I understand it wouldn't be considered a "job" for most people. For me, however, it requires every waking minute to make sure I am giving my body the best opportunity for wellness.

In this job, my body is the boss, and it's a very demanding superior. It demands that I sit before I faint, that I move joints back into their correct location. It demands food it can digest. If I don't carry out any of these actions just as my body desires, it throws an incredible tantrum to let me know it disapproves of my choices. In the life of the chronically ill, our bodies are finicky taskmasters that require constant attention.

I don't always take this job as seriously as I should. Occasionally I make reckless decisions that upset "the boss." Recently I've made questionable decisions regarding using the wheelchair in situations that would otherwise require a lot of walking. I'm always afraid of becoming over-reliant on the wheelchair, so I thought I was making the best health decision. However, to be honest, "the boss" is voicing her disapproval. I'm tired, unfocused, and in pain. I get it, Boss Lady; chill the heck out.

My job is to advocate. I typically like this job. You see, my experience in life is vastly different from many of my peers. I am in a unique position to be able to bring dignity and understanding to the face of disability. I can gently bring awareness to biases and ablest thinking that many of my peers may never have otherwise considered. I'm in a unique position to effect change- where I can.

If I am going to do that, I have to educate myself about my condition. I am not helpful to others if I spread misinformation, so I read medical journals and research reports about Ehlers Danlos Syndrome and Postural Orthostatic Tachycardia Syndrome. I'm not "obsessed" with my illnesses. I don't sit down every night and Google my conditions just to feel more scared. (I don't recommend frequent Googling of anything medical. It'll convince you that you're going to die tomorrow- or that you're already dead!). I research my disorders in order to be the most informed patient and patient advocate possible. The more I know the more I can help to educate my doctors. As a patient with a rare disease (EDS), I frequently meet doctors who have never even heard of my disorder. By being an educated patient, I can guide the doctor toward accurate information sources and ask questions about my treatment as it pertains to my disorders.

One of my favorite things that happens in my new "job" is when I get to meet another person with the same or similar disorders. I have a special love for newly diagnosed patients. I still feel rather lost, but I'll never forget how aimless and confused I felt those first few months. Having a real live person who could look me in the eye and tell me that I can do it would have been priceless. If I can save someone else from that feeling of helplessness and hopelessness (or at least alleviate it to some degree), then I'm honored to have the opportunity to help.

My job is to still be me. It's so easy to lose yourself in illness. In some ways, I'm still trying to figure out who I am now. However, I have a responsibility to my spouse, my family, and my friends to keep being myself. Yes, I am different. Pain changes you. Illness changes you. Fear changes you. I don't apologize for the fact that I'm different from the carefree person I used to be. Having said that, I can still feel the same roles. I listen to and support my loved ones. I love them as deeply as I can. I forgive them when they're insensitive to my illness, and I ask for forgiveness when I'm insensitive to them.

As with all full time jobs, being a professional sick person will sometimes take me away from doing things I would like to do. That's okay too. I know that the first part of my job description is managing my health as well as possible. Now that I know and accept how to do this job, it has gotten easier to forgive myself when I can't do everything- or anything.

A few weeks ago I was feeling especially unwell. I had bronchitis (you know, normal people sick) which had triggered blood pressure problems and dislocated ribs. I felt terrible. I, obviously, can't take a day off from being sick. (A job with no benefits or vacation days? That's just wrong.) I can, however, take days off from anything that doesn't benefit my health.

For a week, I didn't cook, clean, or do anything besides focus on getting better. Why? Because my first job is to care for myself. Did the house get messy? Yes- Joe has the cleaning skills of a college frat boy. Did we eat some weird food? Lasagna and scrambled eggs. That's all I even want to say about that. However, the world kept spinning. The house was still standing. In the end, I eventually got better, and I could get back to some of the less pressing parts of my job description.

If you're like me and you're forever stuck in the cycle of grief from losing your former life, I have a little bit of advice. It obviously won't take the sting away entirely, but it will help you move on bit by bit.

Stay involved with your former field.

As a former middle/ high school teacher, I miss seeing teenagers every day. I don't miss them enough to invite them to my house or anything, but I do miss the interaction. I'm old so I'm fairly lame to hang around with to the average teen, but occasionally I find one that will humor me. I enjoy talking to teens and hearing about their lives. I even enjoy their weird music. (Taylor Swift for life, baby!)

Staying involved with your field is more than hanging out with people like those you used to see. It's also about keeping yourself educated on the changes in your field. I read education articles; I stay up to date on changes in education from a legislative point of view. I read education blogs and listen to stories from teachers in the field now. Does it hurt sometimes? Yes. Do I ache with envy when I hear a teacher complaining about the kid who throws paper or belches all the time (Kids are so strange!)? Every time. But I've toughened up a little. My heart doesn't ache when I see a school bus. I'm not furious every time I hear a teacher complain about writing lesson plans. (Let's be honest- I complained about that nonsense when I was teaching too.) It never quits hurting, but it gets easier. I promise.

Don't isolate yourself.

I left work rather abruptly. I was very ill one day and had to leave early, and then my doctor put me on an indefinite sick leave. Here's where I made my mistake- I never went back to the school. I didn't go back one afternoon and clear out my desk and explain the situation to my colleagues. I didn't return e-mails or phone calls asking where I was. I just disappeared. At the time, I was so embarrassed by all that was happening to me that I felt like I just couldn't handle going back or speaking to anyone. Eventually everyone quit trying. The e-mails and texts ended. The

concern faded. Everyone took the hint that I didn't intend to drop.

Where does that leave me? Mostly friendless. Maybe it would have

happened anyway. Maybe no one could have handled the hot mess I had

become, but I wish I would have let people decide that for themselves. I

spend weeks alone (except for my husband and dog- who are better than

the whole rest of the world anyway in my opinion), and I accidentally

chose it. Of course, I didn't choose to be ill, but I chose to isolate myself

when I was embarrassed by my condition. Learn from my (bad) example.

Keep in touch with your friends. If they want to leave, let them go, but at

least you won't have regrets. Don't hide. You have no reason to feel

shame.

You're allowed to have fun.

Another thing I naively believed about disability is that you have to spend

every waking moment doing "sick people stuff." Here's the thing; I'm sick

every day. I don't need to spend every second making myself more aware

of the fact. Yes, my life stays adequately busy with medicine, doctors,

treatments, and research, but that doesn't mean I don't binge watch "One

Tree Hill" for hours. I used to believe that if I did anything fun I was somehow cheating. I remember being ashamed to meet Joe for lunch,

because that didn't seem like a "professional sick person" thing to do.

(Apparently I though sick people don't eat lunch?)

Do what you're able to do. If you feel like going out for lunch- do it! If you

feel like taking yourself on a picnic- by all means, picnic your little heart

out! (Just watch out for bears, please!) It's no one's concern but yours.

You don't have to hide because you are disabled. Trust me, I hid, and you

know what? No one came looking for me! Get out there and do what you

can. Stay home and binge watch television day and night. Research your

illness. Just keep doing your best to keep moving forward. And, if anyone

has something hateful to say about it? Spit in their eye; you have my

permission.

A Day in the Chronic Life

The point of this chapter is not to tell you how you should spend your days. To be honest, I feel like I need someone to help me schedule and plan my own day. Rather, I want to share a typical day in the chronic illness life with you. Many of you will relate with the struggle and monotony- and others will have a daily struggle far greater than my own.

Wake up #1

This wake up happens typically as Joe comes in the bedroom to shower before he goes to work. This is the first time I come into any sort of awareness of how I feel. Joe showers and reminds me of anything that absolutely has to be accomplished that day. I try to drink water and maneuver my joints back into the correct location before falling back asleep.

Joe is an insufferable morning person. I will never understand his insistence on singing, dancing, and general shenanigans in the morning. I will also probably never appreciate the resulting chaos. However, we all have to do our thing, so I suppose I support his singing and dancing if that's what gets him ready for work.

Wake up #2

The second wake up happens only because I have legitimate "puppy guilt." I have the cutest 11 year old shih tzu that sleeps between Joe and I every night. She would never wake me up to go outside; she loves bedtime cuddles way too much. However, by 9:30-10 I'm aware that my ten- pound ball of fluff needs to do something besides lie in bed next to me. Before I leave the safety and comfort of my bed, I take another huge drink of water and my morning medication.

Then, I go through my getting out of bed process. First, I wiggle my toes to get blood flowing. Then I shake out my legs. Then I bend my knees to my chest. My neck and back are less than cooperative first thing in the morning, so I turn to my side and pull my knees to my chest to stretch my spine. I tuck my chin into my chest and let my neck stretch. Then, I ease my legs over the edge of the bed and try to sit up slowly. (I'm normally so dizzy at this point that I have another drink of water to help with the whole hydration situation.)

Then I set my 4 legged friend, Zoey, in the floor. (It's only fair that I mention that my hands are never cooperative at this point of the day, so Zoey has adapted to me sort of dropping her in the floor.) Then, Zoey and I head out the back door for her to have her morning pee. There are 4 steps between my house and the back gate where Zoey goes outside. I *hate* those steps with everything in my being. I basically waddle down those steps on a wing and a prayer every day. I'm terrified I'll fall- so much so that I always take my cell phone with me in case I end up in a broken legged heap at the bottom and need to call for help.

Assuming I make it to the bottom of the steps without incident, I let Zoey outside. She's easily distracted (or very prone to squirrel chasing?), so I have to keep her on a leash. I have trouble standing without fainting in the mornings- not to mention that standing *hurts*- but Zoey seems to not be phased by that fact. She has the slowest search for a peeing spot ever. I have no clue what she's sniffing for, but I know that it takes my entire capacity for standing in the mornings before she finds her special pee spot. Dogs are weird.

Breakfast

Breakfast is essential as soon as I wake up, because I take medicine and I have a serious fear of ulcers from taking medicine on an empty stomach. However, fixing something to eat when my capacity for staying upright has dwindled is complicated at best. I require coffee- Thank goodness caffeine is delicious, because I need it to get my blood pressure to a decent place. I normally grab a breakfast bar- or if I'm really feeling fancy I fix toast. At some point in *every* breakfast making pursuit, I have to stop and tell Zoey to stop licking herself. (That has nothing to do with chronic illness; I'm just curious if others have the same thing happen.) Then, I carry my coffee and breakfast to the recliner. (Bonus tip- If you have bladder problems, coffee isn't quite as aggravating to your bladder's lining if you add cream. Oh yeah, and cream is delicious!)

Recliner time

I love my husband and all the time I spend with him, but if I'm being honest, my favorite part of the day is my time in our oversized brown recliner. I spend at least an hour eating and alternating between coffee and water. I watch mindless television during this time. (Let's have a collective moment of silence for everyone who has already watched all the episodes of *One Tree Hill*.) I Netflix binge until I come into some awareness of how I actually feel that day.

You see, I feel terrible every day when I first awake. Most days, however, after I move around, have some coffee and water, and eat a little I come to life – sort of. It's frustrating that my entire day to this point revolves around the possibility that I might be able to function- or I might not. However, that's my reality.

Shower

If I'm being entirely honest, some days this is the *main event* of my day. Other days, I don't even make it to the main event. There are a few key questions that happen before I shower. If the answer to any of these questions is "No," I'm at least skipping the hair washing portion of my morning.

Am
"I'm I adequately hydrated to stand in warm water?" (Warm water is a vasodilator, so it can make you faint if you're under hydrated.)

Can I tilt my head back without blacking out? (I don't know why I do this. I'm hoping it happens to someone besides me.)

Is my hair really *that* dirty?

95

Can you tell that washing my hair is a serious struggle? However, one question trumps all others- "Is there any chance of ending up at a doctor's office or hospital today" If the answer to that question is "yes," I'll struggle through a shower, even if I think might not make it.

Getting Dressed

Putting on clothes is an exercise in self-acceptance. Every time I put on clothes I'm aware that my body is falling apart. I'm aware that putting on jeans or a fitted shirt is dangerous- because it might dislocate a joint. I'm aware that I must wear layers, because I sweat like a man and may need to disrobe down to the basics.

Dog Walk #2

I hate to sound like a 10-year-old here, but it makes me giggle that walk #2 is when Zoey gets around to going, um, #2. By the second dog walking, I'm more capable of standing than the first trip. This is when Zoey gets to meander around the house. The desperate hope is that this is when Zoey will choose to have a "bowel performance." Assuming she does, she gets a treat and a lot of attention. (Am I the only person who gives their dog a "pooping cookie" for an adequate performance?)

Errands

I intentionally plan at least one errand per day. If I'm at all capable of driving and existing outside of the house, I want to try it. Some days I don't make it any farther than my car. I drive where I'm going and end up sitting in my car thinking about all the things I should be doing rather than actually doing them. I never attempt long grocery trips- rather I split the week's grocery shopping into multiple small journeys. That is a little frustrating (and expensive) at times, but I have basically *no* attention span so I would never stay focused to get everything. It's easier for me to do a little every day or so.

Besides, I need some social interaction. While it seems ridiculous that I count on the cashier at Kroger for my social experience, it's all I can do. Don't get me wrong- the introvert in me doesn't necessarily want to see anyone, but I still believe it's important to see someone aside from my husband.

Exercise

I try. I really do. I understand that exercise is important to health. However, if I'm being entirely honest, it sucks. It truly sucks to try doing something for your health all the while realizing that nothing is going to fix me. I had a gym membership and eventually realized there was truly nothing there I could do safely. I'm making an effort, now, to exercise from home. Blech. Thank goodness for "Gilmore Girls" or I would never get through a single workout.

Rest

I realize that I slept until 9:30ish, but I require a nap. Normally around the time Joe comes in for work I'm needing a nap- or at least a horizontal resting time. I'm amazed at how much rest my body requires, but I've quit apologizing for it. I'm doing the best I can, and sometimes I have to recharge. There's no shame in that.

Dinner

(Did anyone notice that I skipped lunch? Yeah, my breakfast routine takes so long that I don't even bother with lunch typically.) Dinner is a necessary evil. Joe and I typically cook for his parents when they're unable to cook for themselves. While I'm glad to help all I can, it's so hard sometimes. I want to provide them with a nutritious dinner, and that requires a lot of effort. It's not unusual for me to drop a lot of stuff and dislocate a few fingers in the process.

Joe enjoys cooking- or, more specifically, he enjoys time in the kitchen. He always provides a wonderful iTunes mix while we cook- and a few salty snacks. I have to give him some credit- he helps me cook, but he also helps make the process as much fun as possible.

By the time we finish Joe's cooking countdown of music and dancing (and finish cooking dinner), I'm exhausted. It's not unusual for me to look at my plate and wonder how I can possibly be expected to feed myself due to my level of exhaustion. Fortunately, Joe is very understanding of my desire to always eat while relaxing on the couch leaning on pillows and watching ridiculous stuff on Netflix. I swear, that's the only reason I manage to actually eat dinner and not fall asleep face first in my potatoes.

Mindlessness

The rest of our evening is typically little more than mindless movies and Netflix. Joe has an amazing talent to choose the absolute worst movies on Netflix and insist we watch them. (Seriously, I recently watched "Radioactive Beavers"- an actual movie about mutant beavers- not something as scandalous as it sounds.) I use my evenings to nap (again), catch up on e-mails and social media, and spend some time with Joe. It's not an exciting life, but it's our life. We're happy with it, so I make no apologies.

Bedtime

At bedtime, Joe, Zoey, and I get into our queen sized bed. (Whoever that queen was, she didn't understand the space needs of two adults and a bed hogging shih tzu.) Another night of fighting pain and praying for sleep begins. I typically lie in bed and look at social media until my head hurts too much (from exhaustion I assume?) to continue. Joe is sleeping like a baby. Zoey is snoring like a freight train. I try to find a spot in spite of the space my bed buddies require and sleep. Bedtime is a painful and difficult time of day- but also the time I spend most of my day hoping for. Eventually, I fall asleep, and in a few short hours the whole routine begins again.

The chronic life isn't easy. As a matter of fact, I would gladly exchange it for a day of arguing with middle school students again any time. However, I'm grateful that I'm able stay home and make the best possible decisions for my health. My days are long and boring. There are days that I crave a break from the monotony. Ultimately, though, I have a good life. It's painful- and sometimes boring- but I'm grateful for my family, my

husband, and my dog who make this lifestyle less painful.

Crazy, Chronic Survival Guide to Holidays and Family Events

I have the ultimate love/hate relationship with holidays. They're amazing in theory- time with the people I love most, delicious food, and fun decorations. But, in reality, all of those fabulous things pose a threat to the delicate balance required for a chronic illness.

Time with family and friends also means time in crowded spaces that probably aren't quite large enough to accommodate those gathered. It also means face to face time with family members who don't understand what you're dealing with. Though they mean well, they'll more than likely make you feel awful with their well-meaning sentiments. That delicious food is probably far richer and creamier than my body is accustomed. As a result, I spend most holiday evenings lying in a bathroom floor after heaving into a toilet (Lovely visual, right?). And, the decorations? Geez. I never feel more inadequate than I do at holiday time. Every house around me looks like it could be on the cover of a decorator magazine. My house has a cardboard turkey on the wall or a $20 pre-lit, undecorated tree stuck in the living room. The struggle is real, folks.

Remind yourself that you're the expert on *you*.

Inevitably, someone who doesn't know you very well or know anything about your medical situation will deem it necessary to pontificate on what you should be doing. Listen as politely as possible (They mean well, after all), and then promptly forget their advice if it is in no way helpful to you. You live in your body- no one else does. That makes you the expert. Just because Great Aunt Lulu thinks you would benefit from a deworming doesn't mean that her suggestion has merit or that what you're currently doing isn't adequate. You're the expert on how to live your life and manage your illness. Don't let anyone make you doubt that.

Take breaks.

I always offer to run errands at holidays. What? You need ice? I'm happy to help! Someone needs to go outside and tell people where to park? I'm your girl! I'll be honest; my motives aren't totally altruistic. I need breaks. It's not that I don't love being around my extended family. I absolutely do! However, I overheat easily and get overwhelmed even more easily. A few quiet minutes in the drive way (even if it's bone chillingly cold) help me to cool and calm myself enough to enjoy time with the people I love.

Eat safe foods.

I wish I had taken this advice years ago, but I only put it to practice this past Thanksgiving/Christmas (with 50% success, I might add). Eat foods that you can safely eat. A large gathering is not the time to find out if you're still lactose intolerant- trust me. It's also not the time to try that delicious looking casserole if you know that you don't do well with mixed foods. (I may be the only person like that, but I need all my foods separate prior to entering my body.) At my family events, everyone loves sharing leftovers. If there's a food that you're dying to try but feel unsure about successful digestion, ask if you can take a serving home for later. At least then if your body decides to expel it violently from any orifice, you'll be in the safety and privacy of your own home.

Give yourself a break.

The inclusiveness of holidays is simultaneously touching and disconcerting. I'm touched that my family and friends invite me to multiple events. However, I can't do them all. If I try, I end up miserable by the last one, and I know that's not anyone's intention. It's okay to say

104

no. It's okay to not do everything. It's even okay to show up empty handed or with store bought food. You can't do everything, and the people that love you most will understand that. (It might take some time, but bear with them.)

Christmas and Thanksgiving are beautiful holidays, but neither holiday is about who can do the most. If you're house isn't decorated, it's okay. If your "homemade candy" contribution is a bag of Reese's cups, it's okay. If your idea of gift wrapping is putting the gift in 2 Walmart bags instead of one, it's okay. Do your best, and forgive yourself for the things you can't do.

One of my fears is that I'll become so embarrassed by the things I can't do that I'll quit doing the things I can. I love my family dearly, and I genuinely enjoy spending time with them. As a result, sometimes I have to make some modifications in order to do so. But, you know what? The time I spend with them is totally worth it. Best of luck!

Friendships and Chronic Illness- It's possible to have both.

When I decided to write this chapter, I spent days staring at a blank page in my outlining notebook. I had no idea where to start, because, if I'm being honest, this is an area where I continue to struggle. I have friends, but I'm aware that I'm not the best at nurturing those relationships. It's just so very hard sometimes to act *normal* in spite of illness and general calamity. However, the more I thought about the amazing friends I have in my life, the more I hoped for that support system for others. I hoped in writing this that I was giving others tools to seek friendships- even if they're in a dark place of not being sure friends are all that necessary.

I'm not the most reliable friend. If you need to talk via phone or text, I'm usually available. If you need to meet for coffee and chat, I may or may not be able to pull that off. While I want to be there for you while you're neck deep in marital woes, I might be struggling to stay conscious and not in a safe place medically to drive to you. See, the chronic illness life requires you to be self-absorbed. That probably sounds horrible and selfish, but I have to spend a considerable amount of time thinking about how I feel in order to avoid exacerbating symptoms.

Due to my own self-absorption with my symptoms, I'm always a little confused about how much I'm supposed to tell you about illness. I mean, if we're friends, my health struggles aren't a secret. However, I don't really want EDS to be the obnoxious third wheel at all times. So, in that regard, I'm a little jealous of my healthy friends' normalcy. While every person has their share of problems and friends help share that load, I can't help but feel that no one wants to help share the burden of constant nausea or dislocated shoulder.

So, if having friends is so difficult, is it worth it? I mean, wouldn't it just be simpler to be besties with my remote control and Netflix? Maybe. Maybe it would be easier to be a hermit, but that's not what life is all about. Life is about building relationships. We need friends. If for no other reason, relationships help us to maintain a little bit of normalcy. I mean, if it weren't for friends who distracted me with mindless banter about our favorite books and tv shows, I might spend my whole day Googling my symptoms and imagining the many ways I might prematurely expire. That's certainly no way to live.

One of my biggest struggles has been making friends post- diagnosis. I'm human and innately drawn to that which is most comfortable. For that reason, I tend to depend on my husband and Mom for all my friendship needs, but that's really not fair to anyone. First of all, my husband and Mom can't handle all my drama. Seriously, this hot mess needs to spread out over multiple people. No one can endure all this crazy on their own. It's also not fair to me to not make more friends. If I hide in the safety of comfortable relationships, I will never meet the amazing people this world has to offer. So, I've found ways to make friends in spite of my own insecurities and shortcomings.

Social Media.

The first place I learned how to *be* a human again after getting sick was social media. I was so scared and bitter and hurt by all that happened to me when I became sick that I withdrew into myself for a while. Social media helped me to open up again.

Social media operates on my terms. It is the perfect world for my lifestyle. Social media is 24/7 and happens on my own terms. If it's 3 AM and I'm in horrible pain, someone in the world of social media is awake and willing to distract me from my body's inferno. Also, if I can't handle any interaction for a bit, all social media comes with a log out button.

Social media has its dangers. I realize social media isn't perfect. I realize there is "stranger danger," and there are trolls and catfish and any number of other weird internet slang that means "bad people." I'm not suggesting that you give your address and bank account information to anyone. I am, however, suggesting that social media is a place to reach out for support, and it has been my experience that you will receive the support you need.

Social media can be specific to your needs/ interests. Especially in the early days of your diagnosis, I strongly recommend making friends in chronic illness online support groups. It helps to find others who understand the emotions you're having. I have been beyond blessed to connect with fellow chronic illness friends from all over the world. There are people whom I've never met- and likely will never meet- whom I truly consider friends. I've confided my fears in them. They've helped me through struggles, offered advice, and just read the words I've typed out of desperation when I needed to be heard.

I encourage you to also make non-chronic illness friends. (Because, seriously, it's probably important to remember that everyone doesn't want to hear about your funky rash . . .) Join social media groups for people with interests similar to yours- even if it's something you can't do anymore. If you love horseback riding, join groups for horse lovers. Maybe you can't be a cowgirl anymore, but you can still be part of the conversation.

Real Life Friends.

"Real life friends" are harder for me, and I'm still testing the waters in a sense. I'm learning ways to meet more people and develop relationships, but it has taken a couple years of dealing with illness and learning to accept this life for me to even desire face to face social interaction.

Some friends leave; let them go. You see, in the early days of becoming chronically ill and searching for a diagnosis, I felt really lonely. I don't necessarily believe my friends intentionally left me. It wasn't a conscious decision on their part. Rather, they had no clue what to say to me and, thus, became scarce. It's hard to know what to do or say when your friend's life is falling apart in a way you can't understand or even really imagine. I can appreciate the awkwardness of the whole situation, and I really don't feel hurt anymore that my personal tragedy wasn't met with more support or compassion. (It takes a while to feel that way. It's okay if you're still really angry with the friends who left you.) It's been my experience that those friends eventually return, and then, it's up to you whether you trust them to come back into your life.

Join groups. There are so many groups that seek to facilitate relationships. For example, check with your local hospital and/ or church to see if a support group exists for people who have a chronic illness. If such a group doesn't exist, maybe you're the person your town needs to start it. Join a book club. The great thing about book clubs is that you already know what you're expected to talk about when you get together (assuming you actually read the book). Look at the groups available at your church or community center. Maybe there's a Bible study that appeals to you or a special class. Is there a volunteer organization that would benefit from your help? If so, volunteer and enjoy the new relationships you make along the way.

Be friendly. Ugh. If you ever meet me in real life, you'll think I'm friendly. You might even make the mistake of believing I'm a total extrovert, because at first glance I seem bubbly and talkative. (Okay, at *every* possible glance, I am talkative.) The truth is, however, it really takes a lot of effort and self-reminding for me to be friendly. My natural tendency is to avoid human interaction as much as possible. However, if I want to make friends, hiding and/or pretending not to see people isn't logical. If I see a neighbor out in his/her yard, I challenge myself to say, "Hello." If I meet someone who I hope to get to know better, I force myself to follow up on the conversation- often through social media, because I still feel more comfortable in that world.

Netflix is a vital part of all friendships. Okay, first of all, am I the only person in the world that didn't know "Netflix and Chill" is some weird code for having sex? You've been warned. Do not invite a potential new friend over to "Netflix and Chill" with you. He/she will be scandalized *or* he/she will show up with very different assumptions than you about what is going to happen. Weird slang aside, you don't have to know someone very well to invite them to watch "Gilmore Girls" and eat pizza with you. All the entertainment is handled. All you have to do is laugh at appropriate times, and you're set. It's okay to invite a new friend over to do something totally low key. Every friendship is not built on wild nights out. As a matter of fact, I think most of my friendships are built on fairly calm and caloric nights in.

When I make a new friend, I'm always uncertain about how quickly I should introduce the friend to my chronic illness. Let's be honest, chronic illness is like a really obnoxious toddler- except it doesn't have the redeeming cuteness factor. Because of illness/symptoms, I'm a picky eater, prone to expelling fluids, and a little emotionally unstable. So, it's not exactly fun to drag into any relationship. However, my illness and my symptoms are as much a part of me as my strange laugh or my tendency to talk too much. I've developed a list of guidelines for the introduction of my illness into friendships, because having rules keeps me from panicking about what I'm supposed to say.

Be open (but not obsessive) about your illness. If your days are plagued by symptoms, you're not going to be able to keep that secret. If I go out with a friend and fail to warn them that my joints dislocate at inopportune times, it's going to be a little inconvenient when it happens. (You've not really lived until you've tried to explain your illness quickly and concisely while trying to put a shoulder back into socket.) Let friends know what to expect up front.

Having said that, try to avoid talking about your illness all the time. I get it. Being sick is a huge part of our lives, and we can't escape that reality. However, it's hard to build a relationship with a person when you only talk about one topic. I would never intentionally act as though my struggle outweighs anything a friend might be going through, and I try to keep this in mind when I divulge information about my health.

Allow friends to see you on bad/ flare days. While I think it's important to not bombard your friend with endless statistics about your illness, I also think it's important to allow your friends the opportunity to really be friends. If you're having a horrible day and need some support, tell your friend. If your body is throwing a full-fledged tantrum despite your best efforts to stay well, express that frustration to a friend. Of course, you don't want to do that every day, but it's okay to admit that you don't always grin and bear it. It's okay to cry or be angry at the unfairness of all this. A good friend will commiserate (and a great friend will suggest ice cream).

Return the favor. Great friends are hard to find. If you have a friend that sees you at your worst and loves you anyway, consider yourself blessed. Even though we bring a lot of baggage into any friendship in terms of our illness, any new friend will have an equal amount of issues and he/she will need your support. Be a good listener. Try to empathize with your friends' frustrations. It's hard sometimes, because our worlds are so very different. I have to bite my tongue when a friend complains to me about drama at work, because I miss my own days of being healthy enough to work (and participate in frustrating drama). However, I'm not being a very good friend if I minimize my friend's struggles in light of my own.

Communicate. I truly despise cancelling plans because I'm sick. It sounds like such a cop out. As a result, I sometimes go out when I don't feel like it- or I cancel without an explanation because my explanation sounds lame. Either "solution" to my problem of not wanting to use illness as a reason for cancelling isn't exactly helpful. If I go out with friends while feeling horrible, I'm going to appear moody and miserable- not exactly a fun person to be around. I'll wind up making my friend feel guilty for making me so miserable, and then no one has any fun. If I cancel and don't give a reason, I risk making my friends feel insecure about our friendship. It's easier if I am just honest. I can't do everything. Heck, I can't do a lot of things. I am able, however, to communicate decently. I can reschedule plans or ask if going out to a movie can be substituted by pajama and movie night at home.

Nothing about chronic illness is ever simple. Friendships are no exception. It's difficult to navigate a world that normally involves leaving your house and being social with people that don't understand your private struggle. I understand the complications all too well. However, I'm convinced that humans require connection. We long to feel connected to others. We desire to feel understood and appreciated. Those feelings are difficult to have when your only human contact is at your doctor's appointments. My sincere hope in writing this is that it will give my chronic illness family the encouragement to get out in the world and let everyone see how amazing you are. I don't know about you, but I feel like the world is really missing out if they don't meet us!

Crazy, Chronic Survival Guide to Hanging Out with Healthy Friends

Sometimes I feel like when I was diagnosed I should have been banished to an island with other sick people. Maybe a nice commune of the plagued? I'm joking to an extent, but it really is more complicated than I'd like to admit to hang out with "normal people." By "normal" I mean healthy, of course. I'm not actually sure any of my friends would be considered "normal" by any other definition of the word.

It's just so complicated, you know? Healthy people have no reason to think of mobility, sudden illness flares, or messy bodily functions. Me? Well, it's always on my mind. I'm not being negative; sickness is my reality, and I always have to plan accordingly. Having said that, it's probably not very nice of me to quit being a friend to people simply because they're healthier than I am. So, I've found ways to deal as well as possible.

Make plans. Plans are complicated when you're ill, because the nature of illness is unpredictable. There is always the chance that you'll have to cancel. Friends will understand. Even if they don't "understand," a good friend will give you the benefit of the doubt. Still, if there is a plan in place, I am more likely to attend. I don't do well with spontaneity. Make plans to do something you can feasibly accomplish. Don't tell a friend that you'll meet them at the bowling alley if your condition is made worse by smoke, loud noises, and crowds. I've made the mistake of scheduling something that I could only possibly attend on the absolute healthiest day ever. It's way less stressful to schedule something low key.

Set yourself up for success. I tend to panic in crowds. They're just not my thing. If I'm supposed to do something with a group, I always meet someone beforehand. That saves me the anxiety of entering alone, and my symptoms are less likely to reach a fever pitch when I'm not freaking out over plans. If you're uncomfortable with long car trips, don't schedule a dinner a couple hours away. Do what works best for you. You're not being selfish; you're being realistic.

Keep it low-key. I don't know about you, but I don't think I was ever a partier. I don't have a problem with living it up, but I'm more of a Netflix and nachos kind of girl. I've always preferred low-key nights. Now that my symptoms dictate a lot of my life, I'm much less stressed if I know the night with friends is a calm night on the couch. Of course, low-key can be defined differently for all of us. Maybe you stress over eating with a crowd (I can see how that would be a problem for my friends with very specific diets.). If so, maybe keeping it low-key means skipping dinner and joining your friends for a movie later.

Don't sweat the small stuff. If you have to cancel, no big deal. Reschedule or ask your friend to join you for a movie night if you're up to it. If you get sick while you're out and have to leave, you did your best. Don't stress. Here's the thing- true friends, the people who are worth your time, will be sympathetic. If someone gets upset with you because you couldn't recreate an entire episode of Girls Gone Wild in one evening, maybe it's time to find other friends who can party in a way that's more conducive to you.

Friends are important for this process. One of my regrets is that I didn't do a better job of cultivating friendships in the early days of illness. It's okay though. Friends will stick around, and they'll forgive you when you're not at your best. Do your best; be a friend, and forgive yourself when you can't do everything.

On Faith and Healing

I always hesitate to write about matters of faith. While I am a person of faith, I don't for a moment think that everyone in the world agrees with me. For that matter, it would be arrogant for me to believe that I am right in my beliefs all the time. I'm probably not, but still I cling to my faith as an anchor in a sometimes terrifying storm. I have toyed with the idea of writing this in the wee hours of the morning when sleep wouldn't come. I've always rejected the thought, because how do you write about something so personal? But, as with most things that spark inspiration, this story begs to be told. It has burned so deeply in my heart that it had to eventually be written and shared in some way.

When I first became ill, I believed in miraculous healing. I thought that one-day God would lead me to the perfect doctor, medicine, supplement, or routine that would make my life return to normal. That's not how it worked- at least not for me. I'm not saying I don't believe in miracles anymore. I do. I believe in the miracle of a new child coming into the world. I believe in the miracle of a life being changed by the transforming power of God's grace. I even believe that medical miracles still happen. Surely the same God that raised a man from the dead can fix the earthly maladies that plague us.

However, in all that, I have stopped praying for a physical healing. That doesn't mean when my pain is out of control that I don't pray for relief. I do. I utter many desperate prayers that amount to little more than, "God, PLEASE!" I assume God in His infinite wisdom can fill in the blanks I'm unable to supply. However, I've quit expecting that I'll wake up one day and be "fixed." (Not in the dog sense- in the no longer broken sense . . .)

A couple years ago I was teaching a lesson to children on my Upward team about joy. I was explaining to them that joy was believing that everything would be okay- even when life was going badly. I told them about my own illness and how I had found joy in spite of it. After the lesson and practice ended, one of the children's mothers stayed around to talk. She told me how glad she was that I had been "healed" from my illness. In that same moment, I was leaning against a wall desperately hoping I wouldn't faint while she talked. In all honesty, I had to fight the urge to scoff at her assessment of my situation. In her mind, there was no way I would be working with children, sharing my story, or living a somewhat normal life if I hadn't been "healed." My own reply to her words shocked me.

"I'm not healed- not physically. I have a chronic condition that affects every system in my body. However, God performed a more amazing healing in my life- he healed my heart from anger and sadness and bitterness at all that's happened to me."

It was in that moment that I found my identity as the person I've become as a result of illness. I'm sick, and I'm not happy about it. I don't believe for a second that God gave me this illness to teach me some huge divine lesson. He hasn't made me sick to inspire the world or to show bravery in spite of circumstances. Not at all. I'm sick, because I have faulty genes. However, I'm not angry or bitter about that; we live in an imperfect world and bad things just happen sometime. I don't believe the universe has conspired against me.

Losing that anger is a healing on a grander scale than any type of miraculous physical healing could have been. Pain and illness are hard to endure, but they're not nearly as difficult as living life angry. When I'm angry and bitter I lose the ability to enjoy anything. Pain makes it harder to laugh until I cry or love someone to the point of distraction- but it's not impossible. Bitterness steals all the joys out of life. Ultimately, if I had to choose something to be healed from- I choose no longer being hurt and angry.

I've grown a lot since those early days of hurt and anger, and I'm grateful for that. Part of the growth has come from learning to tune out the pseudo-faith filled messages people share. Some people mean well and have no clue what else to say. Others use their faith as a shield to repel those who need their kindness- rather than using their faith as a net to help the hurting people they encounter. Regardless, I've learned to hear certain phrases, smile and nod, and then refuse to let those phrases shake my faith.

Everything happens for a reason.

Why it hurts: Telling a person that "everything happens for a reason" is cruelly dismissive of their suffering. I'm essentially being told that you offer me no empathy, no prayer, and no grace because my suffering must be for a reason. When I'm told this I feel hurt and invalidated, because you refuse to acknowledge how I must be feeling and instead pile on platitudes that make it sound as though I should be grateful for this mess. I will smile and nod when someone says this. Most are saying this statement because they don't know what else to say. It's fine, really. But, if you have any alternate platitude for the sick and afflicted, please choose another.

The truth: We live in an imperfect world where imperfect things happen. God did not look at me and decide I needed to suffer as part of a grand plan. I truly believe God grieves our pain and heartbreak right along with us. Our loving God- creator of the Universe- does not need me to be sick in order to get His will done. My illness is the consequence of life and the imperfect things that happen to all of us as a result.

God doesn't give us more than we can handle.

Why it hurts: Again, when someone says this, they're essentially saying that whatever you're dealing with isn't less than you can handle. It's a way of trying to cheer someone up by minimizing their struggle- because it hasn't killed them yet. Again, when I hear this, I've learned to ignore it. The speaker might have the best of intentions, but, geez Louise, this is a terrible statement.

The truth: I've already shared my belief that every bad thing that happens isn't God's fault. So, in a sense, God doesn't give us more than we can handle. However, in life exceedingly more than you're able to tolerate will happen. It's in those times that we need faith to help us through the struggle, and we need friends who will be there for us when we can't handle everything alone.

If you just believe and ask God, He will heal you.

Why it hurts: Life, theology, faith, etc- NOTHING is that easy. If all people had to do was believe and ask God in order to be healed, then everyone would be healed already. When someone says this, they're essentially saying that I choose to be sick because I lack faith. While I know that isn't true, it's hurtful to have your personal faith in God called into question as a result of a situation in which I'm powerless.

The truth: I'll be honest; I don't know. I don't know why some people get better and others don't. I don't know why some prayers are answered and others aren't. However, I know that God is a loving God. I know that prayers aren't answered specifically in response to the faith of the one praying. If that were the case, my Momma would have prayed my way to healing years ago- just like so many other mothers in the world who petition God for their child's healing. If you've prayed for healing and feel like you haven't gotten a response, I urge you to remember that you're not at fault and neither is God. I do, however, believe that God answers

125

prayers in His own way. For me, He answered my prayers for healing by healing my soul of bitterness and anger over illness. For you? Well, I don't know, but I believe He's listening regardless.

In what ways does your illness glorify God?

Why it hurts: This question makes me examine myself in a way that isn't helpful. This question makes me feel like however I'm handling my illness, I must be doing it wrong. And, again, questions like this are dismissive of the havoc going on in someone's life. The question says that I can't mourn my illness, because my illness has to be something great and powerful that reflects the glory of God.

The truth: My illness (or any other bad situation in life) is inanimate. It exists without a heart or a soul and, therefore, cannot glorify God any more than an old green truck. Our situations and circumstances are *not* what determine our faith or the practicing of it. I strive to glorify God in spite of illness. That is the best I can offer, but I truly believe it's all God meant for me to give.

These statements (and their equivalents) are hurtful. Often times they aren't meant to hurt, and I try to keep that in mind. If I took these sayings to heart, however, they would wound my faith. I don't want to say the damage would be irreparable, because God is great at mending broken hearts. But, the damage would be severe. As a person of faith who struggles daily with illness, I don't have the time or energy to have the foundations of my beliefs shaken just so someone can offer mindless platitudes. I've learned to ignore a lot. I've stopped pondering over whether or not someone's statement applies to my situation. I've accepted that I'm sick, and my God gives me solace and comfort in the midst of the craziness that surrounds my circumstances.

My goal from the beginning of this book is to offer practical tips to help you through living the chronic life. So, this list is tips to staying in a decent place spiritually when life is a mess physically.

Don't over spiritualize the journey. I've tried really hard not to over spiritualize my journey with chronic illness. While God has been a refuge through times of fear and doubt, I don't want to see every dislocated joint as a spiritual analogy. Eventually, I think that would add to my suffering rather that detract from it. Instead, there are days when I say, "Today just sucked, and I truly hope tomorrow is better" and that's the best I can offer. I am always content with my life spiritually- even when I'm disgruntled physically. God is the keeper of my soul; that's the one part of me I can count on to stay whole. I don't spend my time trying to understand or make sense of all this, because I feel that would be pointless. Rather, I cry when life calls for crying and remember that God will provide me with a fresh tomorrow- and I hope and pray it will be better.

Do your best- and forgive yourself for what you can't do. I was raised to attend church every Sunday (and Sunday night and Wednesday night), and I'm grateful for that. From the time I was a small child, I was taught that if you can be in church on Sunday, that's where you should be. To be honest, as an adult, my church attendance record isn't quite that impressive. However, if I can go- I do. If I'm able to sit up to read my Bible in the evenings, I do. If an opportunity for me to help others presents itself, I do all I can. Life isn't about giving the most- it's about giving your best.

Don't go through this alone. Find a person with a similar belief system and confide in them. Choose a person who will withhold judgment when you rail about the unfairness of this life. Confide in those who show you grace and love when you need it most. Maybe this person is at your church, in your family, your significant other, or a friend you only know through social media. Whoever it is and wherever they are- find someone who can be a physical representation of Christ's love when you're feeling too low to feel that love for yourself. Ask this person to pray for you, and return the favor. Share Bible passages, quotes, and books that encourage you when you're down. Build your own community of believers- even if the community meets through text message or a Facebook group.

You don't have to agree with everyone. I understand that every person isn't going to agree with every word I've said in regard to faith. That's fine. I've been as open and honest as I can be, but I don't assume that just because I feel a certain way that means I'm right and everyone who doesn't agree is wrong. You're going to meet fellow chronic illness sufferers whose beliefs are vastly different from your own. That's fine. I have been blessed by finding friends from different denominations and different faiths who walk this journey with me. I am honored that they pray on my behalf, and I do the same for them.

Being sick is hard, and, at times, it's terrifying. My faith has strengthened me at times when I didn't think I could continue. By the same token, the things that others say regarding faith and illness are at times hurtful- and sometimes just completely ridiculous. It's okay if you don't accept every tired cliché. You don't have to be rude- even well-meaning people say totally unhelpful things at times. However, you also don't have to accept the dismissive things others say as part of your own personal belief system. Do your best, and live your life in a way that best honors the Creator. Oh yeah, and when you totally mess up, don't worry too much. God loves us in spite of our messed-up selves!

Crazy, Chronic Survival Guide- Going to Church

There is no single place that I am more aware of my physical inadequacies than church- which, you know, isn't exactly ideal. It would be super fantastic if church were this wonderful, restful place where I could relax and enjoy the beautiful music and sermon. That, however, is not my reality. Don't get me wrong. I enjoy going to church. I'm a person of faith, and I feel I need fellowship with other individuals of faith for encouragement and growth as a person. I'm not giving up on going to church; I'm simply saying that it is a struggle.

First of all, church is sensory overload. Now, if you have a talent, by all means, use it to glorify God. Hit your drum; bang your cymbals; run the lights and smoke machine if that's your thing. I totally understand that we all have talents, and people want to use their talent to help with the church service. Having said that, holy sensory overload, Batman! Seriously, by the time the music portion of church has ended I'm sweaty and nauseous. The songs are beautiful; to be honest, music is one of my favorite parts of church, but it requires some preparation.

Also, there's the whole standing/ sitting thing that churches and ceremonies tend to employ. I get it; most people get bored from just sitting. Giving the congregation/ crowd breaks from sitting in their pew is probably ideal. Unless just sitting makes your head and neck hurt and the act of standing may very well dislocate your hips or knees. Then, church becomes an obstacle course. (Seriously, could we possibly take lying down breaks instead of standing breaks?) Some religions/ denominations throw in the added even of kneeling . . I admire their reverence, but this girl would never make it through a service. Thank God I'm a protestant; I wasn't cut out for church as an athletic event.

So, what do you do? For me, church hasn't become an impossible obstacle yet. There are things that I do to make it as manageable as possible. It's still an event, and if I'm being honest, there are times I end up watching/ listening to the sermon from home because I just can't do it.

1.   **Prepare for sensory overload.** For me, I know Sunday morning is not the time to eat a huge breakfast. Lights and loud sounds make me nauseous. I always eat something before I go (Adding a blood sugar crisis to the mix sounds like a horrible idea), but I keep it light and bland. Pre-

church toast is my indulgence of choice lately. Also, I look down a lot. If I look directly at the front of the church, the lights and movement are a little too much for me. I've mastered the art of reading my church bulletin intently during moments of sensory overload. I've never tried this, but if you need ear plugs to dull the sound- there's no shame in it.

2.   **It's okay to not follow every direction.** I don't always do all the standing during church when we're directed to do so. I'm not trying to be difficult; I simply assume my pastor would prefer I do what's best for me in order to be able to stay for the entire service. Sometimes I sit during the music. Sometimes I step out and enjoy the music from the foyer rather than listening to it at full throttle. This has occasionally caused an issue. Once Joe sat with me for a moment to see if I was okay on a particularly difficult health day. Apparently a member of the church staff found it offensive. He made his way to us to make a comment about us being "too good" to stand during fellowship time. At that exact moment, it cut like a knife. Within a few weeks,

however, I was able to see his comment for what it was- a misinformed, poorly directed joke. If you're going to be different, you have to develop thick skin.

3. **Don't be too hard on yourself.** This advice is particularly hard for me. Church is important to me. I've gone to every service, Bible study, prayer meeting, and Vacation Bible School since I was a child. Sometimes I'm a little too hard on myself, because the standard was set so high in my childhood. (Don't get me wrong. I'm forever grateful that I was taken to church as a child. I'm glad I have that standard to guide me.) I feel guilty that I can't sit up long enough to go to Sunday school before church. I feel guilty that I don't follow all the sitting and standing directions. I even feel guilty that I can't wear clothes that are as dressy as what I once wore. BUT . . . none of those things matter. I am at church to learn more, to fellowship, to give and receive encouragement, and to be challenged to become a better person. None of those things have anything to do with standing or sitting or wearing pretty clothes. I'm working on this whole guilt thing.

4.   **Reach out to others.** Because of my physical limitations, I lack the sense of community I once had with my church. Everyone is very kind to me, but I can't participate as much as I would like. While I miss being closer with my church family, I have found there are many ways to fill the void of community that are more conducive to my limitations. I participate in online Bible study groups. I have groups that will pray with me and praise with me as well. Of course, this doesn't replace the role of church membership in my life, but it helps me to still have ongoing support when I'm unable to physically be present with my congregation.

I would strongly encourage anyone living with chronic illness to find a congregation with whom they "click." We won't all choose the same type of church or other congregation, and that's fine. However, we all need a source of hope and friends around us to encourage us when we're down.

Crazy Chronic Survival Guide- Surviving a Lifelong Diagnosis

A lot of people, including me, spend years searching for a diagnosis. I have known I was medically different from my peers since primary school. I didn't know what was wrong when I was a kid, and my doctors struggled to articulate what was going on as much as I did. Once my symptoms became so severe that I was forced to address them, I became desperate for a diagnosis- a name to describe the chaos in my body. More than anything, I wanted something that made everything that was happening to me make sense.

I think a lot of chronic illness sufferers spend a while in that trap of desperately hoping for answers that don't come. Then, one day you get a diagnosis. Your doctor orders a test and the results shine a light on the cause of your symptoms. Or you see a specialist who examines you and your symptoms actually make sense to him/her. For most of us, after a long time of searching, we will eventually receive answers. Diagnosis day is a strange mess of emotions. I was thrilled to have a name for what was happening in my body. I felt vindicated to find out that what I have is *real*. I also realized for the first time that I had a lifelong illness.

That was the worst part- realizing that I wasn't going to suddenly get better. A diagnosis doesn't necessarily mean a cure or even helpful treatment options, and the weight of that realization is intense. But, life moves forward with or without me. I had to either get on board and keep moving forward or stay in bed forever. I was scared (a diagnosis also means you can Google your condition and find out about all the lives it has taken); I was frustrated, but ultimately, I was empowered with new knowledge. Getting to a place of acceptance was a process for me, and I imagine it is for everyone. Here are the things that helped me most.

Grieve for a bit. It's okay to take a few days to process how very much something sucks. Seriously. If you need to eat ice cream and binge watch Gilmore Girls for a day or two, no judgment. The people around you may not understand. They may feel like you should be thrilled to have a diagnosis since that's what you've been seeking. Maybe you are thrilled, but that doesn't change that you've just been handed a life sentence without parole. Explain to friends and family that you need a couple days to process. It's not personal, and it won't last forever. It's completely acceptable to sulk, pout, or throw a tantrum.

Find your tribe. You can't stay in bed forever. (Well you could, but I don't recommend it unless it's necessary.) Eventually, you have to reach out to other life sources. I was so relieved to have a diagnosis so I could look for other people like me. I asked my doctors to introduce me to other patients with a similar diagnosis. I joined social media groups, so I could network with others fighting a similar battle. I found support from people who understood what I was going through, and that bridged the gap while I was searching for words to explain what I need to my friends and family.

Seek a fabulous normalcy. Grieving is part of the process. Finding others with a similar battle is part of the process. Eventually, though, you have to move forward. Don't forget the friends you had before diagnosis. Find a way to spend time with them- even if everything feels different than it used to be. Go on dates with your significant other. Watch movies, and laugh until your sides hurt. Your life will never be the same as your peers' lives, but your normal can still be great.

A diagnosis is a great victory and also a great loss. It's normal to mourn the losses, but don't get stuck there. Become an advocate for your disease/ disorder. Fundraise; participate in research; be proactive. Some

of my greatest successes in life have come in spite of a lifelong diagnosis.

Getting a Diagnosis- AKA The Long and Lonely Road

Being chronically ill is hard. It's a lifestyle I wouldn't recommend to anyone. However, it pales in comparison (in my opinion) to being both chronically ill and undiagnosed. Being undiagnosed doesn't mean that you aren't sick- it instead means that you're sick and searching for answers. It means that you don't have a name or even a reasoning to put with the symptoms of illness. The hardest part of being sick for me was the awful time when I knew my body was falling apart and doctors could not give me an answer for the whole mess.

The Struggle of the Undiagnosed-

Disability- Even if you're completely disabled by your symptoms, it's hard to qualify for disability benefits without a diagnosis. Unfortunately, until a judge can see a diagnosis, they have a hard time believing that your illness is real. For me, I was too sick to work long before I stopped, because I couldn't accept that I was disabled by an illness that I didn't even have a name to support. So, I worked as best I could despite my symptoms. I tried to teach all the while taking frequent breaks to vomit, shaking so badly I couldn't write on the board, losing control of my bladder multiple times a day, and being too exhausted to walk my class to lunch (I tried, but I would have to stop to catch my breath along the way!).

Insurance- Insurance companies don't want to cover medications or treatments for an unnamed problem. Needed surgeries and procedures are nearly impossible to get approved. Your doctor wants to try a medication that *might* help (and thus explain some of your symptoms)? Forget it. Insurance companies balk at the lack of information. During the awful years of searching for diagnosis, I had doctor after doctor send me away after he/she couldn't find my problem. They would agree that I was sick, but they were clueless about how to help me. When doctors would send me away, I couldn't get a referral to the next doctor to try to get answers. It was nearly impossible to advocate for myself when my hands were tied by insurance company restrictions.

Symptoms- If you are undiagnosed, new symptoms seem like chewed up puzzle pieces- they don't fit with the picture you thought you were creating. For me, I started vomiting- so I was sent to a gastro doctor. Then I started running a fever- I was sent to a rheumatologist and infectious disease specialist. I lost control of my bladder- I went to a neurologist and urologist. I saw what seemed like every possible "-ologist" the world had to offer, and the list of questions grew while answers never appeared. Here's what no one tells you- most chronic illnesses affect multiple systems. If bizarre things are happening all over your body, there probably *is* a connection.

Validation- I was beginning to question my own mental health. How many times can you receive "normal" test results and still believe that you're actually sick? Doctors suggested my illness might be because I was depressed. In reality, the situation was pretty dang depressing, but I felt like being sick was causing the depression- not vice versa. (It's the whole 'Which came first? The chicken or the egg?' conundrum.) Once I finally had a diagnosis that validated my physical symptoms, I was better able to assess my mental health. During the thick of symptoms, I started to worry that I was imagining my illness- or somehow bringing my symptoms on myself.

Confidence- When I was undiagnosed, I was ashamed to admit no one knew what was wrong with me. I felt like a fraud any time I had to cancel obligations because of illness. My confidence was shattered, and it made me difficult person to be around. (Note- this was in my first year or so of marriage. Lovely, right?) I took medicine that made me gain weight. I took medicine that made me lose weight. My appearance changed rapidly, and I the only thing I had to blame it on was medicine for an undiagnosed problem. I lost a lot of myself during that time, and years later, I'm still mentally recovering.

The struggle is clearly significant. I have friends who have spent decades with an undiagnosed illness, and I truly can't imagine living that way. These same people, however, are some of the strongest men and women I've ever had the pleasure of knowing. I've put together advice from my own experience and others to help those who are pursuing a diagnosis. Granted, these steps won't always lead to answers, but they might preserve your sanity along the way.

1. **Trust yourself.** There will be days when you feel like a fraud. Even though you are fully aware of how terrible you feel, you will sometimes question whether it's "real." Unfortunately, that happens when you receive test after test that show what *isn't* wrong with you and none that show what is. On those days, take an inventory of your life.

Recognize your symptoms and take stock of the sacrifices you've had to make because of illness. No one can fake that. The way you feel is very real, and you deserve answers.

2.   **Be clear with medical professionals.** When I first became ill, I had very limited experience with the medical community. Honestly, up until I was married, I typically asked my mom to come with me to every appointment. I had to learn the hard way that doctors don't just intuitively know everything that is happening in my body. In order to make my symptoms something that could be easily quantified, I began journaling. This was during the years of relentless fever, so I would write down my temperature morning and night. I made note of my pain levels (on a scale of 1-10). I wrote down the length of my menstrual cycle, my bowel movements, frequency of vomiting. I basically had a notebook full of disgusting details about my sick life. Even though doctors probably dreaded to see me and my "poop journal" coming to appointments, it proved helpful. My

doctors were able to look for trends and see the progression of my symptoms by looking at this data.

Also, be clear about how your quality of life is affected. I have the tendency to reply, "I'm fine" any time someone asks me how I'm doing. I, for some reason, feel the need to ensure everyone that I'm doing fine. However, that was completely unhelpful in doctor's visits. I had to learn to be clear and honest about my symptoms and how my life was affected. Saying, "I'm fine, but I've been having headaches" sounds like the headaches are not something I'm wanting to address at this visit. However, saying, "To be honest, I'm having daily headaches, and I'm unable to do daily activities at least twice a week because the headaches are so severe," helps the doctor to recognize this problem is greatly affecting my life and needs to be assessed.

3.   **Advocate for yourself.** Remember how I said my mom always went to doctors' appointments with me before I was married? (Also, remember how I became sick almost immediately after getting married?) I was completely

unprepared to become my own advocate. Yes, I know that's ridiculous. I was 26 years old at the time and a full time teacher with a Master's degree. I should not have been afraid to talk to the doctor, but I was. It took many disappointing visits before I realized I had to be my own advocate. Every doctor isn't prepared to search for answers to medical dilemmas. It's okay to ask your doctor, "Are you willing to help me on this journey?" If he/she is not willing to be part of your search for a diagnosis, find a doctor who is.

4.   **Do your homework.** Okay, there won't be many doctors who will agree with this statement, and that's fine. Search engines and social media are great tools for the undiagnosed. Of course, all this information is to be taken at your own risk. It's not unheard of for Wikipedia to be totally misinformed. It's also very possible that second hand information from someone in an online patient support group isn't reliable. Having said that, we are blessed to be living in a time where a wealth of information is available to everyone. If you're like me, you have plenty of time on your

hands to research possible causes for your symptoms. Of course, your doctor has a medical degree, but more than likely, he/she does not have time to spend hours thinking outside the box. Your doctor also does not necessarily have access to dozens of patients with similar symptoms. Through social media, however, you do.

If you research an illness and think it could possibly bring answers to your situation, mention it to your doctor. Tell your doctor which criteria you meet for the illness. Ask him/her if there is any possibility that diagnosis could fit your situation. Be prepared. There's a very good chance you won't find the answers you're wanting. However, you have at least suggested something new to your doctor that could ultimately aid the journey to diagnosis.

5.   **Build a support network.** This might be even more important than a diagnosis. Find people who support you and believe you. Surround yourself with people who are hoping you find answers. Hopefully, these people will be your family and friends that loved you before you became ill.

Sadly, that won't always be the case. There will be people you love who doubt the legitimacy of your illness. I'm not sure why, but it seems as though it's easier for people to believe you're inventing illness for attention than it is to believe you're legitimately sick. Granted, I feel like their thinking is flawed, but I also feel like if they truly care about you they'll come around eventually.

If you're family and friends can't provide you with the support you need (or if you want to build a larger circle), check out social media. There are hundreds of support groups for the chronically ill or undiagnosed. Of course, everyone in the world isn't an amazing person, but I have been so blessed by the wonderful people I have met through social media. Banish any doubters from your life, and lean on your circle for the support you need during this time of searching.

Being undiagnosed is a daily battle. You battle to understand what your body is becoming, find empathy for an unknown problem, and ultimately just to survive until the day when answers come. Take heart, undiagnosed friends. Every single person will not find a diagnosis, but there's a better chance of being diagnosed today than there was yesterday. Medicine is advancing. Networking is moving forward. Online information is increasing daily. There *is* hope- no matter how dark and hopeless your situation may seem.

Research, Awareness, and Advocacy

Perhaps the best part of being officially diagnosed is being able to find

other patients like me. For the first couple years of being sick, I had no

clue what was wrong with me. I had limited hope for a cure for my

problem, because doctors couldn't find an official name for whatever my

problem was. That era of my life was truly the loneliest and most hopeless

I have ever experienced. I made a vow to myself that if I ever found out

what was wrong with me I would be involved in research and research

funding. I promised I would spread awareness via every type of disease

flaunting merchandise available. So far, I have been able to keep those

promises to myself. If you're looking for ways to be involved with

research, awareness, and advocacy for your illness or on the behalf of

someone you love, here are a few ideas I've tried or plan to try soon.

Research

The only hope any illness sufferer has is a cure or treatment for their

disorder. Cures and treatments are time consuming and expensive, and a lot of people have to be willing to sacrifice in order for breakthroughs to happen. I have had the unique experience of participating in research for Postural Orthostatic Tachycardia Syndrome (POTS), and I am so very grateful for those opportunities.

Research has allowed me to dialogue with some of the top doctors, researchers, and other medical professionals in the world for my condition.

The very first time I participated in a research study at Vanderbilt Medical Center I was terrified. I had only been diagnosed a few weeks, and I was searching for answers. When I checked into the inpatient research facility at the hospital, I was greeted by nurses who were used to patients like me. I quickly met doctors who were the best in the world in treating my illness. The took time to explain the purpose of their research and findings from previous studies. Research doctors often have more time to answer patients' questions than doctors in a clinic. This allowed me to get advice from those who were most knowledgeable about my disorder within weeks of diagnosis. I don't doubt that the treatment success I have had is due to the early advice I received from top doctors.

Research has allowed me to meet other patients like me.

When I went to Vanderbilt the first time I felt truly friendless. I lacked the words to explain what was going on in my body, and I felt like no one truly understood me. Within the first couple days of being at the research facility, I met Lacey and Leslie. Both of these wonderful ladies also had POTS and understood my struggle. They encouraged me to live and laugh again. We wandered the halls taking ridiculous selfies and gagged over the five gallon buckets full of slimy peaches that were served with every meal. These ladies have been part of my network of support since the day we met. I still text them if I have an illness related question- or a ridiculous meme- to share. Meeting people who could empathize with my struggle validated and empowered me to become the person I am now.

Research gives me hope.

Every few months, new research regarding a disorder I have is released. Sometimes the research confirms something doctors already suspected. Other times the new information opens researchers' minds to new opportunities for a possible cure- or at least a treatment. As a patient, I find so much hope in the fact that there are people who spend their days trying to help patients like me. Researchers are my heroes, and I'm so grateful they're willing to go into the trenches with patients to help us find answers.

Research is expensive.

There are dozens of diseases and disorders at present that are without any type of treatment or cure. While there are certainly very intelligent doctors, pharmacologists, and other researchers who may be able to find answers, their work is expensive. Not only do all the medical personnel involved need to be compensated for their time and effort, there is also the expense of lab time and equipment, medication expenses, and countless other details. While government funding for medical research exists, there is not nearly enough to cover the extensive research needed to find a cure for the thousands of rare disease sufferers that deserve answers.

As patients, we can help fuel progress by donating and fundraising for the research organizations closest to our hearts. For example, I take online surveys frequently. As the money accumulates, I donate it to Dysautonomia International or The Ehlers Danlos Society. My donations are small; they typically happen in $10-20 increments. However, I'm doing what I can to be part of process of finding a cure. I have limited talents and skills, but I use those I have to raise money for research. Other ideas I've tried or considered include selling awareness ribbons in my disorder's awareness color(s). Most people are willing to dole out $1 toward disease research- especially if they get a cool ribbon or sticker to show they helped!

Awareness

I catch a little bit of grief for spreading awareness. I understand why. To people who have never had their life thrown in the spin cycle by sudden illness, I probably seem obsessed with being sick. I'm not. I do my best to forget as often as possible. However, I owe it to the chronic illness community to use any platform I have to spread awareness. I'm not obsessed with illness; I'm committed to informing the world about my disorder. The truth of the matter is if I had *any* awareness whatsoever of what chronic illness is my transition to disabled life wouldn't have been so painful. I had no idea that people became sick and didn't recover. I should have known- I had family and friends with chronic illness- but no one was talking about it.

The amazing part of spreading awareness of an illness is when someone you know finally gets answers to their own health concerns based on the information you've shared. If I had met even one person in the Ehlers Danlos Syndrome community before my symptoms became so overwhelming, I would have sought medical attention and perhaps have avoided the fallout of symptoms. That didn't happen for me, but I hope that I am that beacon for others looking for answers.

How do you do it? How do you spread awareness for a disorder without walking around yelling, "I'm sick with x, y, and z!" (That will probably land you in quarantine- you've been warned!) There has to be a least obnoxious way to spread awareness, right?

Know your awareness month.

You know how there are a lot of really stupid holidays like chocolate pudding day? Well, occasionally our society's desire to celebrate everything pays off. Most (if not all) diseases and disorders have an awareness month. For an entire month, you're actually expected to share information about your illness. How cool is that? Most disease foundations have graphics on their social media platforms that you can share. This is also a great time to tell your personal story. Post a video and get real with your friends about your struggle. This is the time to let others know what you're going through. Fair warning- be kind always.

Raise awareness. Share your struggle. Don't belittle others because they haven't been through your struggle. (Even if they are complaining obnoxiously about a head cold or another ridiculous ailment.)

Also, I like to make my awareness months (May for Ehlers Danlos Syndrome and October for Dysautonomia/ POTS) a pseudo- Christmas. I tell Joe I require an awareness month gift. I don't *actually* expect a gift. Rather, I post something silly on social media every time he buys toilet paper or Diet Coke thanking him for the awareness month gift. I'm fortunate that my husband doesn't mind me picking on him a little for the sake of awareness.

Find allies, and build your tribe.

I became strong and empowered in the world of chronic illness by finding others like me and leaning on them for support when I couldn't stand alone. When it comes to spreading awareness, partner with a group who shares your illness and take over social media. Tweet celebrities, politicians, or others with a large social media following. You may only be able to reach out to a few people on your own, but with a group your voice gets louder. When you work with others to spread awareness, your cause becomes bigger. The truth of the matter is money for research happens when those with power and finances become aware of a problem. The more people that are spreading awareness- the more likely you are to get your need in front of the right people.

I have met a lot of people through blogging my experience. The more I share about my struggle, the more I found out I'm not completely alone. My first blog garnered a measly 30 views, and I thought that was amazing. Despite the low activity, I made new social media friends as a result of sharing my experience. As I wrote more, I met more people. Eventually we formed an online support group that not only supports each other- but we spread awareness for the illnesses of other members. My blogging experience has landed me on sites that I would have never dreamed would pay attention to me. I've met new friends through being published on The Mighty and Global Genes. To be honest, I'm still blown away that my tribe has expanded in such amazing ways, and I'm thrilled that I have had the honor to spread awareness on very respected platforms.

Be creative.

Remember the ALS Ice Bucket Challenge? I'll be honest, I thought it was nothing more than a social media phenomenon. Nope. Legit money was raised and donated. How cool is that? Some person poured ice water over their head; someone else thought that was hilarious, and then there was a social media takeover that resulted in a lot of money being donated toward ALS research. That money funded breakthroughs in research! Now, we don't all have ALS, but we all do ridiculous things like pour water over our heads to entertain our friends. We all have the capacity to use our creativity to raise awareness (and maybe even money) for rare and/or chronic illnesses. Who knows? You may play a role in the cure for AIDS because you start the "Wear your underwear outside your clothes" challenge. Use your creativity; use your gifts. Play the kazoo for Keshan disease. Pole dance for Paget Disease. Yodel for Charcot Marie Tooth. Do what you do- and do it to raise awareness.

Advocacy

Is it strange that I'm a little scared of the word "advocate"? It sounds so angry to me. I immediately imagine a person holding a sign and screaming obscenities. I'm not that person. There is truly nothing angry or confrontational about me (except when Joe forgets to put the new toilet paper on the roll- then the situation gets heated). I'm learning, however, that it is okay to confront the world about the injustices that exist for the disabled. As you become more aware of your own limitations, you also become more aware of how inaccessible the world can be to the chronically ill. I'm embarrassed that this wasn't on my radar before I experienced it, though.

It is perfectly acceptable to speak up on the behalf of others who are oppressed. I realize we don't automatically think of the chronically ill as being oppressed, there are times when our society doesn't show nearly enough empathy. Medical care has room for improvement- in spite of being the profession of many brilliant and caring individuals. Disabled accessibility is improving thanks to ADA laws, but there is still room for improvement. Just because we are sick doesn't mean we don't expect the world to be accepting of us. We have a voice, and we can be heard. We aren't a bunch of sick people- we are advocates for our entire community.

Use your gifts.

Use your talents to advocate for the disabled community. Please. Do it. I can't draw anything – except a marginally acceptable hippo. I can't sing. I can't play music (much to my mother's chagrin- who paid for 6 years of piano lessons). I am a decent writer, and I thank God that my gifts have developed in a way to speak about the life and challenges of the disabled. Whatever you do well- use it as a way to speak up for yourself and others.

Speak on others' behalf.

I could spend my whole life speaking about the injustices that I face, but what is the point in that? I have friends and family who face larger challenges. If I do not use my voice- in whatever limited capacity I'm granted- to speak up for them, then I have missed an opportunity to help someone else. Whatever you choose as your way to advocate for others, use it for someone besides you. Don't get me wrong. I expect that we will all rail against the injustices we face personally. However, I also expect that we will weep with the weeping and rail against the injustices that face our other chronic illness family.

Act in love- not anger.

It is okay to be angry about unfairness. It's perfectly acceptable to be mad that about discrimination, oppression, and lack of awareness. I understand, and I'm right there with you. However, strive to act in love. When your heart breaks because a friend couldn't watch a movie because he/she could not gain access to the theater, respond with kindness. Love your friend. Object injustice. Act kindly. I understand the desire to yell and scream, but we're better than that. Write a letter. Post on social media.

Passively and lovingly explain that *every* person deserves to be able to access public areas- not only the physically capable.

Believe me. I understand the desire to angrily advocate on social media or in person. I understand the intense desire to set others straight- especially when they seem to be discounting those who suffer physically. I implore you to act in love. It's perfectly acceptable to be angry, but do not let it influence how you act. Act kindly. Rather than call them out in an angry manner, remind them that not everyone is blessed with the health they have. Explain the struggle you and others face. Ask others to empathize. If they are incapable, then remind them you are protected by the disability law. But, please, save that reminder until you've tried empathy first. Advocacy is best shared kindly- I promise.

Ultimately, research is driven by the advocates. Awareness is necessary for funding- and our own validation. My own experience in advocacy and awareness has taught me that love always wins. Through becoming an advocate of my disorder and chronic illness as a whole, I have met new friends, gained new influence, and realized a new purpose I could have never imagined.

Victim vs. Advocate

There are the early days of illness. Maybe you were born with your illness and symptoms, so you don't know life without being sick. For me, even though I was technically born with my genetic anomaly, the symptoms didn't take over until I was an adult. So, I had a sudden realization of symptoms, and in those days, I was a victim. I was the injured party in a series of unfortunate events. It is probably pretty normal for those of us who live the disabled life to suddenly have a realization of "This sucks!" or "Why me?" In the early days of illness, everyone is a victim. A victim (according to Websters.com) is a person who has been attacked, injured, robbed, or killed by someone else; someone or something that is harmed by an unpleasant event (such as an illness or event). Am I by definition a victim of illness? Yes, absolutely. However, I choose to be more.

What is the danger, though? If I am a victim of the wrecking ball of illness what is the harm in owning it? For me, I feel if I accept the identity of victim I become too focused on the bad things in life. I become too focused on the way I don't measure up to the standard of others. I recognize that my life didn't pan out the way I expected, and I never move past that grief. Becoming a victim is too painful. If I'm a victim, I'm less likely to spread a message of hope- I run the risk of spreading discouragement and fear, and I'm not that person.

An advocate (again, as defined by websters.com) is a person who argues for or supports a cause or policy; a person who works for a cause or group; a person who argues for the cause of another person. If I have to choose a personal identity, I choose advocate. Would I rather be a person who is always bemoaning the ways that life has kicked me in the face or would I rather be a person who is standing in the gap and working for a cause? The choice is easy. I'm not a victim anymore. I'm an advocate.

I have to remind myself of this frequently, or I slip back into victim mentality. Don't get me wrong. There are days when I feel horrible, and my body is falling apart more quickly than I can pick up the pieces. On those days I have victim moments. I have days where I cry and wish desperately that my life had taken a different path. However, I don't get lost in that identity. I take a few days to mourn my losses and keep moving forward. I remind myself that I have fought too many battles to stop fighting now. Sure, there are struggles and "victim moments," but ultimately, I choose being an advocate.

I have to educate. As an advocate, I choose to educate others wherever I go. I don't strive to bore others with details of my illness. Instead, I tell others about the community of chronically ill and disabled friends I have met through illness. I share about the amazing people I've had the opportunity to meet within our community. I share about our needs and struggles. I encourage others to join me in standing in the gap for all those who are ill.

Advocates have a different way of looking at struggles than victims. Advocates are working for others- for a cause or group. Victims are fighting a personal battle; advocates are fighting for all of us. When I face challenges regarding chronic illness, I ask myself how I can best advocate for not only myself but all my chronic illness friends. How can I argue for the cause of my entire community?

With difficult people

If Taylor Swift has taught us anything, she's taught us that in life you'll meet haters and doubters and people who are just plain mean. As a chronic illness patient, you'll meet perfect strangers who feel it's their job to comment on the veracity of your illness. You'll meet doctors who are rude or dismissive to your needs. You'll encounter friends and family members who find you much too high maintenance to keep in their lives. You'll meet difficult people, and you'll have to decide how to respond. It's only fair that I tell you that my first reaction is to be a victim when I'm faced with adversity. If you've reacted as a victim in the past or do so now, don't be too hard on yourself. We're humans.

Victims- Victims respond by reminding others all they've endured. They lash out. They feel crushed by the lack of understanding being conveyed and respond with anger. That's normal. If life has treated you unfairly, it's natural to want to share the depths of the injustice. The problem with this response is that it doesn't accomplish anything. When I react to difficult people with anger, they don't hear what I have to say. The difficult people believe that their behavior was justified- because obviously I'm an angry bitter person rather than ill. See what happens? In our efforts to justify our illness, we can give other ammunition to continue to judge us unfairly. (Granted, difficult people will more than likely judge you unfairly regardless. They're frustrating like that.)

<u>Advocates</u>- Advocates stand up for themselves and others like them by educating difficult people. If a doctor refuses to listen, an advocate says, "I don't feel like you're listening to my concerns. Are you uncomfortable treating my condition?" When a stranger makes an inappropriate comment, advocates say, "I have a chronic illness that causes me to look/ act differently. Would you like me to tell you more about it so you won't unfairly judge others like me?" When a family or friend complains about the effects of our illness on their lives, advocates say, "I understand my illness affects you as well, and I'm sorry about that. Would it help if I explained why I need additional help?" Advocates speak up and speak out against injustice; however, advocates also know that in order to get others to listen, they need to speak with grace and kindness- not anger.

During a Symptom Flare-

Anyone living in our chronic illness world knows exactly what I'm talking about. You wake up one morning, and you can't sit up without getting dizzy. Or suddenly your pain levels go through the roof. Maybe you run a fever or vomit everything you try to eat. Whatever your flares are like, they all suck a duck.

Victims- Victims shut down during a symptom flare. They can't imagine

how life could get any better. Victims believe that a bad day equates a

bad life. While I realize we all have those moments, victims do not move

beyond them. Victims add to their own suffering by believing that the

suffering will never lessen. The grieve their losses before they're gone.

I recently dislocated a few fingers after an evening of coloring (Adult

coloring books are dangerous, kids). The next morning, I was convinced

that I was losing the use of my hands. I spent my morning crying because I

can't type on social media. I worried that I would never be able to blog or

write again. I was drowning in my losses and hopeless that the situation

could improve. I eventually realized that I don't require working fingers to

type. There is a voice to text feature on my phone. There is software that

will type for me on the computer. I even have a husband who will type for

me when I can't. When the victim part of my brain slowed down, the

rational part of my brain reminded me that my life wasn't over.

Advocates-- Advocates go through the victim mentality more than likely.

It's hard not to feel like victim when you're tossing your cookies a dozen

times a day. However, advocates remind themselves that life can and

probably will get better. Advocates contact their doctor and ask for help.

Advocates reach out to others with a similar diagnosis to see if they have any tips to handle any new symptoms (Don't try anything new without asking your doctor, please!). Advocates do their best to keep moving forward and maintain hope- even when life is being particularly painful.

Spending Time with Others-

Spending time with friends and family is a legitimate struggle in this lifestyle. While I love being around people who mean a lot to me, it's uncomfortable. I feel like I'm going through inspection to see how much my health has deteriorated. I feel awkward when I'm not capable of doing something my healthy peers are able to do. These situations have to be approached with caution, or I run the risk of making those I love most feel unimportant or disregarded.

Victims- Victims are very aware of everything they can't do. When I'm being a victim (yeah, I'm not always an advocate), I can give you a list a mile long explaining why I can't do anything. I can't go out with friends, because sitting up will give me a headache. I can't invite anyone to the house, because I don't feel like cleaning. I can't go on a date night with my husband, because I don't even have the energy to wash my hair. While all of those are valid reasons why I can't do things sometimes, there are days when I *can* do things- even if they require more work and effort than I want to put forth. Victims sometimes forget that those they love are worth the effort- even if it's hard.

Advocates- Advocates realize that they represent all those in their illness community, and they want to represent them well. As an advocate for the chronically ill, I find a way to get out of the house and put forth every effort to spend time with those I love. There are days when symptoms prevent me from doing anything, but if there's a way to make it happen, I make it happen. Sometimes that means I use a wheelchair. Other times it means I change plans. Regardless, I'm the face of chronic illness/ disability for many of my friends, and I want to represent us as positively as possible. I'll probably never be able to spend an afternoon at a trampoline park or rock climbing gym, but I'm always down for some Gilmore Girls binging and raw cookie dough. (Egg free- I'm not an animal!)

Awareness-

Victims- When you're a victim, you feel like you have to constantly convince others that you're sick. This is partially a side effect of dealing with difficult people, so I understand the proclivity. Victims tell those around them about every bump and bruise and headache- even if they're not medical professionals or caregivers. Victims feel the burden of proof for their illness- regardless of the fact that their illness is very real and doesn't require evidence.

Advocates- Advocates share information about their diagnosis (and others' diagnoses) in hopes of helping undiagnosed friends find answers. Advocates help others brainstorm ways to find a qualified medical professional who will help them. They understand that their illness is real and doesn't require any verification. However, they gently and kindly share information about their diagnosis with medical professionals and others in order to increase understanding for others.

The truth of the matter is there's not an exact moment when you become an advocate. I haven't had a life changing experience that suddenly made me stop being a victim. To be honest, I have victim moments almost daily. However, I'm learning to shape my actions and reaction based on how I want to represent the chronic illness community. It seems to be human nature to be a victim when bad things happen. If you catch yourself slipping into victim mentality, that's fine. However, remind yourself that you are capable of being more. You're capable of being someone who advocates for all those who have been victimized by illness.

In all fairness, it's easier to be a victim. Being an advocate is exhausting. I've explained the same things to the same people many times, and it's exhausting. Some people are resistant to my gentle education, but I think it's fair to expect more from our society. I expect everyone to continue to learn, and if it takes me multiple tries to teach someone about my diagnosis or the disabled community as a whole- that's okay. There will be days when you won't have the energy to do all that, and I understand. I'll advocate for us when I can, and on the days I'm too tired, I hope you'll stand in the gap for me.

I want to be an advocate for myself and for the disabled community. I want to temper my responses to adversity to convey strength, resilience, hope, and kindness. My goal is to weather this chronic illness storm with as much grace and humor as possible. By doing that, I hope I'm showing newly diagnosed sufferers that their life isn't over. Life with a chronic illness is hard. It's unfair; it's disappointing. However, it isn't a sentence to a life as a victim. There is life after diagnosis, and I've found that life through finding my identity as an advocate for others.

Body Image and Illness- I make broken look good

I feel like one of the great consistencies in my life is my body doing the exact opposite of what I requested of it. I say, "Go!"- my body refuses. I say, "Think!"- my body draws a blank. I demand that my body digest a meal, and it responds by violently expelling food at the least opportune of times. My body pulled the ultimate betrayal when it became sick, and it continues to remind me daily that it refuses to behave. I'll be honest, the whole situation irritates me. Even in those terrible and awkward middle school and early adolescent days I wasn't more aware of my imperfections than I am now. I feel like I'm stuck in perpetual adolescence. My body is forever changing and doing new, unexpected things, so it's hard to feel at peace with the way I look.

Even more difficult is the realization that I feel powerless to do anything about my body's many shortcomings. Illness tattoos your body. The longer you're ill the more illness imprints itself upon you. At this very moment, I'm very aware that I could stand to lose a few pounds. Various medications have made my weight fluctuate, and I'm beginning to exceed the expectations of the elastic in my leggings. My eyes look sunken and dark. I've started leaving sunglasses on in pictures so I don't look like I'm living in an abusive home. One of the many weird things that EDS does to your body is to cause easy bruising and stretch marks. I get stretch marks and bruises from a joint that frequently dislocates until my skin resembles a map. Today, my joints are extra swollen. The last time I looked at my knees I noticed they bore a striking resemblance to Lord Voldemort's face. If that doesn't scream sexy, I don't know what does!

This is just the short list of imperfections that I bemoan. There have been horrible days where I stared at myself in a mirror (Yes, I realize I might have a bit of a struggle with vanity.) and told myself repeatedly how disgusting I am. I was exhausted from fighting a battle that I didn't feel strong enough to endure. I was frustrated that my bladder was choosing to act at the least convenient times possible (Unless you consider a crowded movie theater a logical place to relieve yourself . . .). I was disgusted by the tired, sick, and weak woman I saw looking back at me from the mirror. Of course, telling yourself how gross you are doesn't really help anything. While I'm all for going through your personal process and doing all you can to move toward acceptance, at no point was it beneficial for me to berate myself. Especially as a female, the world will tell me all the ways I don't measure up; I don't have to add insult to injury by self-humiliation. In spite of all that, I continue to be my own worst critic.

Despite all my flaws, there are still many things about my body in which I feel pride. I'm still alive, and I've had to fight to get to this point. Now, I'll grant that I haven't had too many life threatening situations, but every day has been a battle to get to this point. In spite of the wreckage that is my body, I am still trying. I am still working on this somewhat broken body, and I'm proud of that. Lastly, the marks I wear as a result of illness are not marks of weakness. Sure, they're a constant reminder of the ways I'm less than normal, but they're also a reminder of all that I continue to overcome.

Niceties aside, though, how on earth do you ever accept and learn to love a broken body? It's hard. There are still days that I act like a 12-year-old trying to figure out what to do with her newly acquired breasts- except I'm 31 and trying to figure out how to cover up newly acquired varicose veins. But still, there has to be a way to remain confident while stuck inside a body that insists on reminding me that it's broken.

Go back to Sesame Street.

Do you remember watching Sesame Street as a kid? (Seriously, it's the only reason I can sort of count!) One of the things we learned as small children watching "Sesame Street" was that it doesn't matter what people look like on the outside; it's what is on the inside that matters most. While that seems to be the theme of most children's shows, adulthood quickly teaches us otherwise. If you watch children playing, they are drawn to the kids that are kind and share. They're drawn to kids who want to go on great adventures to the top of the monkey bars with them. They don't care what they're friends look like. However, as adults, we begin to believe that there is more value in those who look perfect. We grow up and at some point replace the truths we learned as children with the myth that only the beautiful have worth. I am certainly guilty of second guessing my own worth because I feel less than confident with the way I look. Here's the truth- our broken bodies are simply rickety houses for beautiful hearts. We are strong, courageous, kind, funny, and so many other things that matter infinitely more than having perfect skin or toned abs.

Work on the person you are on the inside first. I've found that a lot of times when I'm embarrassed by how my exterior looks it's because my interior needs some work. While I can't heal my body of illness, I can work

175

to learn more; I can meet new people who challenge me to be better. I can love more and laugh more and try to love the person I am- even if I have reservations about the person everyone sees on the outside.

Do whatever gives you confidence.

I realize it seems counterintuitive for me to suggest a beauty routine immediately after discussing why the way we look doesn't matter. If you're perfectly confident wearing nothing but your underwear, by all means, go for it. (Be warned- most places require a bit more clothing than that. I'd at least carry around a pair of pants for such situations.) While it doesn't matter how you look- how you feel about yourself certainly matters. If there's something that makes you feel more confident, indulge to whatever extent you can. For me, I hate my pale skin. I think it makes me look especially sick- not to mention the bruises and stretch marks really stick out in contrast to my skin's milk-like hue. I spray tan as often as I can afford. It's entirely possible that I look like an Oompa Loompa at all times, but I don't care. The fake pigment covers up the dark circles under my eyes and the bulging veins on the back of my legs. I'm more confident when I'm able to camouflage some of the signs of illness on my body.

Maybe you don't care about spray tanning, but there is some other indulgence that bolsters your confidence. If you're at all able, I encourage you to do whatever helps you feel better about yourself. Maybe that means you take an evening to do your nails. If so, go for it! Maybe you have to splurge for a massage or facial because that will make you feel more self-assured. Don't beat yourself up over it. You're doing the best you can to manage an extraordinarily difficult situation. If you need a mud bath to deal, may your mud time be a reminder of how very much you've earned a little pampering.

Comfort is Key.

My tolerance of uncomfortable clothing has definitely dwindled since I became sick. There was a time when I could feel perfectly confident in shoes that pinched my toes and an itchy dress. Now? I'm doing well to hold it together in sweat pants. I honestly make an effort to look as nicely dressed and appropriate as possible, but I am not willing to put up with uncomfortable clothing as part of that process. If I wear uncomfortable shoes, I spend more time worrying about falling than I do realizing how cute my shoes are. Nothing wrecks your confidence more than worrying that you're about to take a face dive every time you step. Dress in a way that doesn't hinder you. I once met a lady that mentioned she felt uncomfortable always wearing pants to church, but she was afraid to wear a dress because she fell frequently. My advice to her- and to all of us- is to do what works for you. If she tried her luck wearing a dress or skirt to church, she would spend all her time worrying about accidentally flashing the congregation if she stumbled. Do whatever makes you most comfortable- societal norms don't really matter.

Make clothing and style decisions based on what works for you. Maybe physical comfort isn't your concern so much as the type of clothing that is the least hassle. That's fine too. I hate wearing clothes that I have to constantly adjust, for example. Seriously, I spend half my day adjusting my joints' position in their socket; I don't need to spend the other day making sure my skirt covers my behind. Make decisions based on what makes life most accessible and available to you- not on what a magazine says you're supposed to wear!

Everybody is insecure.

I grew up with beautiful friends. I didn't choose them because they were beautiful. Somehow, though, when we all went through puberty, puberty was kinder to my friends than me. While I struggled with my braces and glasses and frizzy hair (Seriously, what was I thinking with those perms?)- my friends had perfect hair and teeth and, to my knowledge, never had a pimple. Is that an accurate reflection of what really happened? Not at all, but I didn't know that at the time. As a teen, I was convinced I was a hot mess, and all my friends were pictures of perfection. It wasn't until we reached college and adulthood that we started talking about our pubescence, and I realized everyone felt the same way I did. We all felt like we were the mess of the group and everyone else was gliding through puberty with ease.

What I've learned as an adult is that everyone is very aware of their flaws. The person you watch and assume she would never have a reason to doubt herself is more than likely as plagued with insecurities as you are. Come on- you know that girl. Even today, as an adult, you know someone that seems absolutely perfect. There is that girl that appears to be so beautiful and perfect that you imagine she never sweats- or passes gas. Here's the truth- we're all worried about how others perceive us. We all fear that someone is going to look at us and see all the ways that we're inadequate. The good news is that everyone is so busy worrying about their drama that they hardly have time to notice what is going on with you.

Your significant other loves YOU.

The place where I struggle most with insecurity is in my relationship with my husband. In my mind, there are million better choices for a wife than me. Every day I have moment of realizing how much better he could do if he really wanted. Couple that with my insecurity about being alone and sick, and you have a serious lack of confidence. None of that is Joe's fault. He has never held me to the standard to which I'm measuring myself. However, I'm forever aware that I'm not as pretty, or as active, or as thin as so many other women I see.

In spite of my worrying, the fact remains that my husband chose to marry *me*- not someone else. He knew when we were married that eventually I would age; he probably assumed it would take longer than it has, but still, he chose to marry me in spite of the fact that he knew I would someday have wrinkles and white hair and adult diapers. When I'm really being honest with myself, I am aware that I chose to marry Joe because I love his heart and his brain. I think he's handsome and attractive- and he still makes my toes tingle when he kisses me. But, ultimately, I wanted to marry him because of who he is rather than how he looks. I take solace in the fact that he seems to have married me for the same reasons. He loves me- not the way I look (which is great since that seems to vary from day to day).

Remind yourself how incredible you are.

There will be days when you feel disgusting. There will be days when you're aware of everything mark of illness on your body and not able to see beyond that. That happens despite your best efforts to prevent feeling that way. On that day, look back at all that you've battled. Realize that every bump and bruise you see is proof that you made it through a struggle. Remember that you are strong and resilient and those qualities matter way more than a thigh gap.

There will be days when you don't have the energy to care what you look like. That's fine too. If it took all of your energy to get a shower today, then congratulations on showering. If you don't have the energy to lift your head off the pillow long enough to even shower, that's okay too. I promise; you're not gross. You're fighting a battle, and you need all the rest you can get to recharge for the next fight.

This is one of the most difficult areas of chronic illness for me. I'm ashamed by how much my life revolves around my insecurities about how I look. However, in the deepest part of my heart, I'm aware of a few key truths. I have fought too hard to live in spite of illness to allow my insecurities to cripple me. I will probably always be acutely cognizant of the ways in which my body could use improvement. However, I'm not going to miss days on the beach with nephew and niece or nights on the town with my husband because I'm insecure. I'm better than that. Illness has made me too strong to act like that. I challenge you to enjoy your life- and stop worrying about the imperfections you imagine are blatant.

Caregivers as Romantic Partners

I sort of hate the term "caregiver." It's so ridiculously broad. When I refer to a "caregiver," I could be referring to a home health aid or a significant other. The caregiver's role could extend to all basic functions (feeding, mobility, toilet issues) or it could be simply providing transportation and helping the sick person out of the floor when he/she falls. It's a complicated term, because while it sounds very sterile and institutional- it could refer to one's own romantic partner. Sexy, right?

I, at times, refer to my husband as my caregiver. He drives me to appointments. He sometimes has to help me stand up or walk down steps. He does the things in our house that my body will no longer allow me to do (taking out trash, mopping, moving/ lifting objects). At other times, I'm the person who has to match his clothes (Poor guy. He was born with terrible matching skills.), so in a sense, he's the one receiving care. When you're married (or in a long term relationship) with the person who acts as your main caregiver, the lines are blurred.

It's only fair that I admit my caregiver experience (as an adult with chronic illness) is solely based on my husband as my carer. It's possible that every caregiver/ care receiver dynamic is equally as confusing. I don't have adequate experience to make a judgment regarding that. From my experience of having my significant other double as my care provider, I've realized that there are some ways that this is not an ideal relationship dynamic.

Sometimes, it's humiliating. In a regular relationship, you're never going to call your partner and work and ask them to pick up super absorbency incontinence pads, because you're afraid that if you leave home you'll make puddles. Does that make me feel like a disgusting beast? Heck, yeah. Joe and I have had so many embarrassing conversations that it is ridiculous. We try to keep boundaries. For example, Joe never walks into a room when I'm using the restroom. (Obviously, he would if I needed him, but we haven't gotten to that point.) He doesn't need to witness the world of pads and catheters and general feminine hygiene. He knows it all exists, but, for now, I'm content to keep the clear boundaries in place.

There's so much guilt. If I'm being entirely honest, Joe does more than his fair share. He works during the day, and when he comes home he's met with the demands of whatever I can't do by myself. I feel horrible that he has so many extra responsibilities. In a relationship where both partners are healthy, there are set expectations for both people in the relationship. However, expectations keep changing here. One week I might be perfectly fine to do the laundry. The next week I'm dealing with dislocating hips and can't walk downstairs to the laundry room. I feel guilty every time I need to add something else to Joe's already sizeable to do list.

I'm demanding- or at least my body is. A background joke in many sitcoms involves the wife asking the husband to do something and the husband replying, "In a minute, honey" (or some similar response to stall). In my relationship, however, when I ask Joe to do something, I normally need immediate action. If I ask him to set a pan out of the oven, it's because my arms won't lift it. There are times when I'm already holding something before I realize I actually *can't*. Then, I'm yelling like a maniac for Joe to come help. Sometimes, my need for help is immediate, but Joe's response is not. I end up coming off as demanding or mean. It's never my intention, but, if I'm being honest, pain and fear can make me a little irrational.

A caregiver fault does not equate a relationship problem. I have to remind myself of this quite often. There are times that Joe is not as sensitive to my needs as I wish he would be. I end up hurting myself because he didn't anticipate my need and offer help. If his job was 100% caregiver, then maybe that would be a failure on his part. However, his job first and foremost is to be my husband. He never wants me to hurt. He would never try to hurt me. If something doesn't go as smoothly as it could, that doesn't mean there's a problem with our marriage. It could mean that I need to communicate my needs better. It could mean that he needs additional help in dealing with my needs. It, however, does not mean that he doesn't love me or that he isn't trying.

This life isn't sexy. It's just not. What no one tells you when you get married is that life is never as black and white as your wedding vows. When Joe and I vowed to love each other "in sickness and in health" we thought it would be one or the other. We thought the line between being sick and being healthy would be clearer. That's not how it works. There are a whole lot of in between days. It's not poetic; it's actually considerably less poetic than a "normal" marriage. Our lives are messy and complicated, because both of us are playing roles we never imagined ourselves having.

However, in spite of all the difficulties, there are things we can do to make this role easier for each other. I have learned that there are Dos and Don'ts receiving care with as much kindness and grace as possible.

Dos for receiving care from a significant other-

1.   *Be kind always.* Remembering to say please and thank you goes a long way when someone is dedicating their life to your care. Even if the dinner your caregiver made is burned or smells like vomit, appreciate the effort.

2.   *Communicate needs.* If someone has assumed the role of aiding in your care, you have to tell them what you need. The other day, I was frustrated with Joe for not taking the trash out. I tried doing it and managed to pop my shoulder out of place. In retrospect, if I had asked him to take out the trash instead of angrily doing it myself, I could have saved both of us some grief.

3.   *Do more than say, "thank you."* Don't get me wrong. It's great to say please and thank you. The basic rules of politeness are a good place to start. However, if you say that you're grateful for help but never show that you're grateful, the words will lose meaning. I thank Joe for his help, but I also continue to do the

things I am capable of doing to help him. I do nice things for him to let him know his efforts are appreciated.

4.   *Maintain as much independence as possible.* I can't begin to explain how tempting it is to ask for more help than I actually require. There are certain tasks that I *can* do, but it hurts to do so. That's okay. If the pain isn't detrimental to my overall condition, I endure it to maintain independence. Walking down my patio steps in order to walk the dog is slow and torturous. However, until I am physically incapable of making it down the steps without injury or incident, I will continue to walk Zoey. Would it be easier to ask Joe to takeover that responsibility completely? Heck, yeah. But, for now, that isn't necessary, and I don't want to require more assistance than I must.

5.   *Recognize that I still have a relationship role.* I am not solely the receiver of care in this relationship. I am a spouse, first and foremost. That means that while Joe meets my physical needs by driving me to appointments or helping me stand up, I meet his needs by listening, helping, and encouraging. I still have a role in this relationship. I minimize extra work by organizing

tasks that must be done. I help Joe with portions of his job that I can do (like brainstorming new ideas, typing lecture notes, or putting grades in the computer). I listen to his ambitions and frustrations- even when those frustrations are a direct result of his role as my caregiver.

Don'ts for receiving care from a significant other-

1.   *Don't be snarky.* I'm sure this will come as a great shock to many of my readers, but I can be a bit of a smart aleck. As a matter of fact, I think I'm more fluent in sarcasm than English. It's a gift, really. However, when someone is taking time out of their day to help me, that is definitely not the time or place for me to share my "gift."

2.   *Don't feel like you must prove your illness.* This has been a legitimate struggle for me. Joe has never made me feel like he doesn't believe my illness is real. (Granted, he's been to doctor's appointments with me, so he has a basic idea of the reality of my illness.) However, there have been other non-believers that have left me feeling insecure about my disabled status. As a result, I sometimes fall into the trap of telling and showing Joe everything

that is wrong with my body. The harm doesn't lie in oversharing about your illness. If you *need* to talk about it, that's fine. For me, the harm was that I felt like I had to prove the legitimacy of my illness to the person whose opinion mattered most to me. I was entering conversations defensively- when I didn't need to defend anything. Joe, on the other hand, was left tip toeing a line where he was trying to keep from saying the wrong thing.

3.   *Don't expect your significant other to be a professional caregiver.* If you happen to be married to a person in the nursing field, this might be different for you. However, Joe is a college professor. If my illness required that he present research and lecture to a group of students or colleagues, he would be well equipped for that task. However, my illness requires him to do things for which he hasn't been trained. No one taught him how to help me get out of bed. Sometimes that means he hurts me more than helps me in the process. He was never trained in pushing a wheelchair in a way so as not to injure the rider. Again, he struggles with this. Sure, he's learning. However, neither of us expected my life to be the way it is. Thus, neither of us were prepared for our current reality. I've had to keep my expectations

reasonable and remind myself that my husband is learning this lifestyle with me.

4.   *Don't stop trying to be romantic.* This is hard. I feel about as attractive as a rotten potato most of the time. I can't imagine how my husband still loves this weepy, leaky mess. However, I try to be loveable. I dress in nice clothes (as much as I can tolerate) when Joe and I go out together. I send him texts to let him know I'm thinking about him. I make every effort to show that I am still very much in love with him.

5.   *Don't minimize your partner's life.* My life can seem like the hottest of messes sometimes. My days are filled with constant reminders of pain and illness. It's easy to get so absorbed in my own problems that I forget that Joe has his own issues. However, I am only one half of a relationship. My problems and concerns are not the only problems that exist for us as a couple. If Joe is concerned about a problem at work, that is equally as important as my dislocated shoulder. Yes, physical pain is *loud*, but it's important that I not treat my problems as more important than

my partner's. (Although, reason prevails, and I typically reset my shoulder before I ask about Joe's day.)

I've said it before, but it bears repeating- This life isn't sexy. There's nothing glamorous about asking your husband to leave a restaurant because your bladder just spewed its contents on your jeans. There are awful moments of having your husband find you lying on the bathroom floor drenched in sweat and reeking of vomit. This is hardly what either of us imagined when we signed on for "holy matrimony." However, we are finding ways to make this life work for us as well as possible- despite inevitable bumps in the road.

When the Normally Healthy Partner is Sick- AKA The Grand Apocalypse

Have you heard of the "man cold"? It's a grave illness unlike any ever contracted by a female. The man cold renders the patient incapable of even the most mundane tasks- putting a glass in the dishwasher, putting toilet paper on the roll, or in severe cases, picking his clothes up off the floor. It's a grievous illness- the likes of which I have yet to experience. I imagine if I were to give natural birth to a 10 pound baby while simultaneously passing kidney stone and having an organ rupture, I might understand the depths of pain my husband feels when he has a cold, or a headache, or tummy ache. Maybe.

Of course, I'm being facetious. Joe isn't that terrible when he's sick. Actually, if he's truly, legitimately sick, he's the model patient. He once had a horrible stomach virus that cued an episode of fainting and landed him in the hospital. He was such a trooper through that whole experience. But, geez Louise, if he gets a headache, his world is on fire. There's weeping, wailing, and gnashing of teeth- and that's just when I make him take a Tylenol. Fortunately, he's rarely sick. I can probably count on one hand the number of times in our almost six year marriage that he has actually been ill. I, on the other hand, have been sick a lot. Joe is fantastic at helping when I'm sick. He does tasks for me that I'm sure he never imagined he would have to learn to do. Based on his track record of helping me when I'm sick, he deserves all the empathy in the world on the rare occasion that he isn't feeling well. But, oh my goodness, the drama! There's some serious drama that accompanies his every ailment.

There are several issues at play when my normally healthy spouse is sick. He despises going to the doctor. He will complain about a symptom but refuse to go to the doctor. I am so used to going to doctor's appointments that I have a hard time comprehending why someone wouldn't seek medical intervention. However, since Joe isn't accustomed to how being sick feels, everything is frightening and overwhelming. Going to the doctor just adds another level of anxiety to his already sickened state. If I'm being entirely honest, being temperamental is normally my role in this marriage. I have a hard time with the role reversal. My empathy skills are not what I want them to be when Joe is sick, and it's something I should make a conscious effort to improve.

I have a picture in my mind of the type of wife I want to be when Joe is sick. I want to return every favor he does for me when I'm unable to carry out everyday tasks, and I want to do those tasks without snarkiness (a serious feat for me). I want to be a selfless caregiver that models the kindness I receive when I'm sick. I would love to be able to show my appreciation of all that Joe does via some mad nursing skills.

However, in all reality, I won't be that person. Instead, I'll be irritated that he won't go to the doctor. This sounds horrible, but I have a compromised immune system. I have to be concerned that I'll catch whatever funk he's carrying into the house. I know that it's awful to be worried about catching someone else's illness when he's in the throes of suffering, but I know that a simple cold can wreak major havoc on my body. Also, I'm still sick. Even though Joe is acutely sick, I have a chronic disorder that I am trying to handle while nursing him back to health. So, in spite of his weakened state, I'm limited in how much help I can offer him. I still can't lift the trash from the garbage can. I still can't walk down the steps to the washing machine at times. I can't even run errands for him until I'm properly medicated. Amid his illness, I'm still walking the tight rope of my own day to day condition.

None of that reasoning gives me an excuse to be a less than sympathetic caregiver. While I may not be able to fully understand *why* Joe feels the way he does, as his wife, I still care that he is in distress. I compiled some tips to help other chronic illness friends cope and help with the role reversal when the typically healthy spouse/ caregiver is the sick. I'll be honest. Most of my tips were discovered by me doing the exact opposite.

A bit of advice for when your normally healthy spouse (or partner) is sick .. .

Remember, your partner isn't accustomed to feeling poorly- this really feels like the end of the world to him/her. For those who don't live with chronic illness, being sick is an event. It feels like period of mourning. I know, I can't fully understand it either. While a headache or stomach upset is background noise for those of us who live chronic illness, it is a memorable event for someone who does not live that way. This doesn't mean that he/she is weak or whiny (okay, maybe a little whiny). It means that this is something new and unexpected to your spouse. Remind yourself of how you felt when you had a new symptom. It's frightening, and you have to train your body how to handle it. Your spouse is going through that adjustment. More than likely, your spouse will get better, and this new illness will never become background noise for him/ her. However, I'm guessing if these symptoms stayed, he/she would figure out how to handle them eventually- just as you've learned to handle your myriad of symptoms.

This isn't the time to be passive aggressive- or just plain aggressive. Of course, it's never a good time to be passive aggressive toward your spouse (or anyone for that matter). However, I feel a distinct temptation to be difficult when Joe is sick. When he asks me to bring him something, I want to sigh and act like it's a burden, so he knows how I feel when he does that. There's a very immature part of me that wants him to appreciate my sickness and the accompanying struggle while he's suffering with his own medical issues. There's even a part of me that wants to cram every tiny mistake he has made in the past six months into the one afternoon he has a headache. Yes, it's immature, and I typically don't actually do it. However, the temptation is there.

I have to remind myself that one of my spouse's roles in our relationship is being a caregiver. Therefore, just as with any role you play in life, he makes mistakes. (And, to be fair, sometimes he doesn't make mistakes- rather I have some perceived slight that didn't exist) It's hard for anyone to get it right all the time. If I have a problem with something Joe is doing or is not doing, it is my responsibility to talk to him about it. More than likely, it is a misunderstanding. It is *not* my responsibility to passive aggressively "give him a taste of his own medicine." No one is helped by such childishness, and it could ultimately lead to more serious relationship problems.

Do your best, and that's all you can do. On the flip side of all the admissions I've made regarding my lack of empathy when my husband is ill, there's also a part of me that feels guilty when he's sick, because I want to be able to do more. It stinks when he's sick, and I still can't open a can or a bottle by myself. I truly hate asking him to get out of bed or the recliner to carry laundry up the stairs, because I can't do it. However, I am honestly doing my best. As long as I am doing all I can to help as needed, I'll forgive myself for the rest. Sure, it would be nice if I could manage everything by myself, but Joe lives with me. He's used to all that my life requires. I will listen to his needs. I'll provide him with meals and medicine. I'll run all needed errands as much as I am capable. I will do everything within my limited capabilities for him.

Ultimately, I will always struggle mentally and physically when my spouse is sick. I fail to fully appreciate the depths of his suffering at times. That's my fault, and I'm working on it. However, in marriage and relationships, you do the best you can and realize that you won't be perfect. Joe and I weren't prepared for our lives to be as complicated by (my) illness as they are; however, when we chose to be together we were committed to facing life together. If that means I have to nurse Joe through a "man cold" while I'm standing on a dislocated hip, I can learn to deal.

Medical Anxiety- AKA Meltdowns of Epic Proportions

As I'm writing this, I'm in a season of higher medical anxiety than normal. I'm awaiting results from a test that could change my entire diagnosis/ prognosis, and living in the land of uncertainty makes me a nervous wreck. I keep repeating that I refuse to worry until I know that it's time to start worrying. However, the truth is that my mind is somewhat preoccupied with fear of the unknown.

While I feel justified in my current level of concern, I also must admit that I have a certain flair for the dramatic. A few weeks ago, I woke up and noticed that my dog, Zoey, had something dark matted in her fur. It looked like blood, and I immediately switched into panic mode. I called Joe at work and told him I might need to take Zoey to the vet. I asked him roughly three dozen questions about whether he had noticed Zoey acting unusual lately. I gave Zoey a treat to see if she acted as energetic as normal. (She did. She *always* has energy for a treat.) I searched her fluffy body to try to find the source of the bleeding. Then, I noticed a sweet smell- almost like molasses. My hands were sticking to her fur. Upon sticking Zoey in a tub of water to further investigate, I realized she wasn't covered in blood- she was covered in barbecue sauce. I still don't exactly know how it happened, but I know she was never in any danger. The "near- death" doggy illness turned out to be nothing more than a need for a bath and a bit more supervision for the canine.

Is it ridiculous that I panicked over barbecue sauce on my dog? Yes, of course it is. However, in that one awful moment of noticing a potential problem with Zoey, my mind immediately jumped to every worst-case scenario. My tendency toward drama is exhausting at times. I joke that most my exercise comes from jumping to conclusions. In all honesty, my actual response was tempered compared to how I felt on the inside. In my mind, I was terrified. I wanted to cry and rush my dog to the vet. The truth of the matter is that I can make a potentially bad situation into a pressing disaster by the time I have mentally processed it.

Obviously, I'm not exactly proud of this aspect of my personality. At the same time, though, I don't apologize for it. It would be nice if I were the type of person who could stay completely calm at all times. But, if I'm being honest, my past has taught me that under reaction is just as dangerous. I would rather process the worst-case scenario and accept its possibility than be surprised by an outcome far worse than I could have imagined.

This is especially troublesome in regard to chronic illness. I have lost friends with the same diagnosis as me. That reality tends to make me fearful that every new problem is life threatening. There are days when I start to worry that a simple muscle ache is a blood clot. Is that a little ridiculous? Absolutely. But when you live with a serious diagnosis it's hard not to imagine that everything that happens to my body is serious as well.

Here's a confession I've never told anyone- after a small aneurysm was found on my carotid artery, I started writing letters to my nephew and niece. I was so afraid I wouldn't be around to see them on important days in their lives (graduations, wedding days, spiritual milestones) that I wanted them to have a piece of me with them for those days. I realize that I'm being a little dramatic; it's not like I was given a terminal diagnosis. However, fear can make you do unusual things.

However, in spite of all this, I know one thing- I have to do better. I truly want to do better; I really do. I realize I will always be a drama queen. (If you don't believe me, you should listen to my dramatic retelling of the time I met Honey Boo Boo.) I have to find a way to reign in my fear and the resulting meltdowns, because if I don't, I'm going to waste a lot of 'good days' worrying about "what ifs." Not to mention, it's really not fair to those closest to me to have to listen to me discuss not only my actual medical problems- but also all *potential* problems. I have implemented a few positive changes that have helped me cope better now than I was before. I'll share those changes, and I hope they help you learn to manage on your own medical anxiety. I don't want to make the leap of saying you should follow my example, because, honestly, I'm sure there's someone out there that shows far more grace under pressure than I do.

I stopped reading medical reports repeatedly. You know what I love? Patient portals. I love that the internet has made it possible for patients to be active and informed in their own care. I always read my lab and test reports after they are posted on patient portal. This helps me form questions to ask my doctor, and I value my role as an informed patient.

However, patient portals became a detriment to me, because they allowed me access to my medical information any time I felt the urge. I ended up reading reports from last brain scan in the wee hours of the morning (when I'm too exhausted and in pain to be rational). I was Googling out of range lab results any time I was feeling anxious. I told myself that I was being proactive, but, in truth, I was fueling my anxiety. I have had to promise myself that I will not check patient portal unless I need to know an appointment time or if a new message or report is received. I won't read my doctor's notes multiple times and try to decode an implied meaning (that probably doesn't exist in the first place). I won't read through reports and Google each term and how it relates to my diagnosis. I read the report; I talk to my doctor. That's it.

I acknowledge my fear. I have a serious problem with lying to myself. I'm a pretty convincing liar too. I tell myself that I'm not scared. I convince myself that the only reason I am talking about potential health concerns is to help others be prepared for what could happen next. But I'm lying. The truth is that I'm scared, and I can't form a thought or conversation without mentioning my fears. By convincing myself I wasn't scared, I was stuck in a loop where I couldn't talk about what was really going on in my head.

I notice I'm less anxious when I call fear exactly what it is. When anxious or obsessive thoughts take over my brain, I admit those feelings are fear. Fear is easier to address when you recognize it. If I'm feeling afraid or anxious about a medical issue (or life in general), I will admit to myself

204

that I'm scared. I'll talk to my spouse or family about my struggle with fear. Normally, once I've talked about it and allowed other people to help me, the fear and anxiety aren't so bad.

I distract myself. Obviously, this isn't professional advice. I understand that a problem doesn't go away by ignoring it. However, if I've already admitted to myself that I'm scared, I don't see the point in making myself dwell on my fear. So, to the extent of my ability (and to the extent of Joe's ability, because he is the great 'planner of fun' around here), I find other things to think about. I watch dumb movies. I watch all the seasons "Gilmore Girls" for the hundredth time. I download new apps for my phone that will entertain me when my mind would normally have time to wander. (I highly recommend Logic Puzzles and Disney Emoji Blitz. Those are my current favorite apps when I need a distraction.)

From the onset of my illness, Joe and I have found ways to make the best of difficult situations. We go shopping after doctor appointments, have date nights after tests, and plan trips when we're in a season of waiting for results. At the moment, we're planning our annual trip to Disney World which will take place just after I receive the results that I'm feeling anxious about. Knowing that I have something to look forward to, allows me to look past my fears and see the fun that is coming. Of course, that doesn't guarantee that I won't receive bad news, but it does mean that life will go on regardless of the outcome.

If I'm being entirely honest, my system isn't perfect. I have moments and entire days where I worry more than I wish I would. However, I'm making an effort to take back some of the control that fear has over me. My best advice to anyone who also feels overwhelmed by anxiety and fear is to keep trying to overcome it in whatever way works best. Find a distraction. Talk to a friend or family member. Speak to your doctor about how anxiety is affecting your life. Give yourself permission to acknowledge that being sick is scary. And, realize that you're not alone in handling that fear.

Letters to Those Who Don't Understand

I can't be the only person who gets really irritated by the lack of understanding and accessibility for the disabled and chronically ill in our society. Now, these aren't things that are eating me alive or that even keep me from enjoying myself. However, there are tons of tiny annoyances that no one would notice unless they're mobility challenged or otherwise physically limited. So many times I've longed to explain to a store clerk, event staff, or random people I encounter how a small change would greatly improve my ability to enjoy an event or outing. Of course, I don't want to be *that person*. I don't walk around expecting people to accommodate me and my hot mess of a body. However, there's an inner dialogue going on that I'm dying to share. So, I created the final section of this book- a group of letters to address the minor annoyances. These letters will never be distributed (at least not by me), but I'll share them with you because I believe you'll understand.

Dear Church,

I know that the church isn't a place that needs to receive my criticism. So, please understand, this comes from a place of love and intense desire to make everyone's worship experience as accessible as possible. I write this not to criticize but, rather, to let the church body know how some are affected by the words and actions of the church service.

Let's start with general accessibility. Look at your church building. Is there a way for the disabled to safely access the rooms where events are held? Are the accessible routes labeled so that those with disabilities who are visiting can most easily navigate the building? Is the elevator or lift clearly labeled (directions of where to obtain the elevator key, if necessary; instructions of who to call for assistance)? Is handicapped parking sufficient and safe? Are the pathways from said parking sufficiently cleared of ice/ snow in inclement weather? Are in-home Bible studies occurring at homes that are accessible? If not, are participants adequately informed of this beforehand?

These are the questions that I wish someone was asking. I know that churches aren't trying to exclude the disabled or differently abled. However, the truth of the matter is that I often feel like I can't participate due to the unknowns related to accessibility. I'm not proposing a total overhaul of events; I am suggesting a little more awareness of the situation.

Next, may I suggest slight changes to the language used to direct worshippers. For example, "Let's all stand and sing" seems innocuous enough, but if it were adjusted say, "Please join me in singing- and stand if you choose" then those like me who can't stand for a ten-minute worship through music session won't look as though they're choosing to not participate. Several times in the past few years since my symptoms have worsened, I've had other worshippers comment about me sitting during the music portion of church. I assure you that I'm not choosing to not follow directions. I am simply incapable of standing for that long without causing more distraction than necessary. (Trust me, if I faint during church, it will cause a greater distraction than me sitting while others are standing.) Again, I don't think that churches use language like this to make others feel uncomfortable. They simply do not realize that others' abilities are different than their own.

Lastly, I think it would help if the church would open their doors to support groups for the chronically ill and disabled. According to the CDC, almost half of all adults suffer from a chronic health problem. Of course, every person isn't affected to the point of disability, but the fact of the matter is that roughly half of adult parishioners are struggling with their health daily. Rather than demean their suffering by telling them they have to be happy in spite of circumstances (which you don't; the Bible clearly shows that God hears and understands our suffering), let's address the suffering through prayer and support. Of course, every chronically ill adult won't feel the need for such support, but for many of us it would be helpful.

Again, I don't think the church is trying to alienate the ill and disabled. I simply feel as though there is room for growth and improvement. From the bottom of my heart, I appreciate the love and acceptance for all people that is shown in many places of worship. It's because of that love and acceptance that I feel confident enough to ask for more.

Thank you for your time.

Peace, love, and health.

Dear Mean Mugger,

I see you. I see the face you make when I park in a handicap spot (with a legally obtained handicap parking permit). I see the eye roll when you see my list of medication at the doctor's office. I'm very aware of the wide-eyed look you give me when you hear that I am disabled. I'm almost fully immune to dirty looks and scoffs at this point, because I've seen them all.

I don't judge you for the look you give me. If I'm being honest, my face reacts to situations sometimes when I would prefer it not. More than likely you don't intend to be hurtful with your 'mean mugging,' so I'm going to give you the benefit of the doubt. However, I want to explain a few things to you, so you will understand my situation. Maybe your face will behave the next time it witnesses me doing something that doesn't seem "normal" for a healthy looking 32-year-old.

I am sick. I am sick every day. I am sick enough that my doctors have deemed me incapable of doing the job I trained and studied to do. You see, chronic illness is different than the typical illness experience. When a healthy person gets sick, the sickness lasts a finite amount of time. One day you're sick, but in a few days, you'll be well. Since you're sick for a limited amount of time, you can take a time out from life during the time of your illness. For me, sickness works very differently. I am sick. I don't have a sudden, acute illness that only last a short time. My illness is part of my everyday life. As a result, I can't take a day off from responsibilities until I feel better. I run errands while sick. I go on date night with my husband while sick. I even go on vacation while sick.

I understand your confusion. I really do. I realize that my life is very different from yours. All I'm asking is that you consider this from my point of view- and the point of view of the many chronically ill or disabled people throughout the world. Getting out and doing things we enjoy is very difficult for us. Please, reserve your eye rolls and scoffs for something that actually deserves them. I mean, there are people who kick puppies.

Roll your eyes at them. People who blow their nose (loudly!) in a restaurant? Scoff at them. Leave me and my chronically ill friends alone!

Thanks for your time.

Peace, love, and health.

Dear hotel staff,

I have a strange relationship with hotels. I stay in hotels a lot. It's not that I particularly enjoy sleeping in a bed that has been slept in by hundreds of strangers in varying states of cleanliness. As a matter of fact, the thought makes me shudder. However, my health has reached a point where day trips are almost impossible. Riding in the car causes me a lot of pain, so if I go somewhere more than an hour away, I have to spend the night to rest before the ride home. I tell you all that to say that staying in a hotel is not a luxury experience for me. It's not a vacation; it's a necessity. There are certain tweaks you could make to the hotel experience that would make my stay easier.

First, if I have reserved a handicap accessible room, please don't feel like you need to assess my disability status upon check in. Don't feel like you need to ask, "So, do you need a handicap accessible room?" Seriously. Why on earth would I have gone through the trouble to reserve an ADA room if I didn't actually want it. Furthermore, if I have reserved an accessible room, please do not make changes to my reservation without notifying me. I get it. Things happen; people overbook. I am completely understanding about mistakes. However, if I am going to be showering in a shower without rails or a seat, I need to bring slip resistant shower shoes, electrolytes to ensure I won't faint from dehydration in the heat of a shower, and maybe some dry shampoo so I don't have to bother with washing my hair. Again, situations happen, but a 'heads up' would be very appreciated.

Next, please pay extra attention to the cleanliness of an accessible room. Those with disabilities typically have a compromised immune system. Do you know what isn't exactly ideal for compromised immune systems? Varied bodily fluids. So, if said fluids have stained the shower chair, sheets, and toilet, I don't exactly feel safe in the room. Everyone makes mistakes. Cleaning staff can't be perfect regardless of how hard they try. I understand that. However, please take extra time when cleaning

212

accessible rooms. Clean the grab bars in the shower. Clean and sanitize the shower seat (You would not believe how many times I've found hair or excrement on a shower seat.). For those of us who require such things, we are at your mercy to provide us with clean and safe facilities.

Lastly, let's talk about electrical outlets. This doesn't necessarily apply to my situation, but a lot of my friends with disabilities need outlets near the bed for medical equipment. I realize that you can't create outlets where they don't exist, but it would be helpful to maybe hang a sign that informs guests that extension cords or power strips are available for medical needs.

I'm not a difficult customer. I will gladly give you a great online review if my stay is remotely comfortable. I don't expect you to jump through hoops to please me. However, I am making suggestions that would make the stay of many guests more pleasant.

Thanks for your time

Peace, love, and health.

Dear Social Media Merchant,

Congratulations on your newest business venture. I am so excited for you as you take these steps to offer greater financial support for your family. That is commendable. I realize when you work in multi-level marketing sales and advertising are done through social media. Hey, there's nothing wrong with that. I've used my social media account for Netflix recommendations, recipe ideas, and even the occasional restaurant suggestion. I can appreciate the myriad of uses when you have the whole world at your fingertips.

But . . . let me ask you a favor. As you begin your business, go ahead and promise yourself that you aren't going to become a vulture. I get it. You're confused. How could selling green pills or purple drinks possibly turn you into an opportunistic vulture preying on those with illnesses? I'm not entirely sure how it happens, but I know it's a very real risk. Let me explain.

If I post something on social media that is intended for my chronic illness friends and I use a hashtag like #chronicillness or #chronicfatigue, I will be suddenly bombarded by new "friends." By friends, I mean people who will start following my account, because they are searching those tags. Are they fellow patients? No. Are they offering support or prayers for those who have those conditions? No. Instead, they have learned that if they pitch whatever unapproved health product they're peddling onto people who are suffering they are tapping into a desperate group of people. While the ill and disabled rarely have a lot of expendable income, they are often desperate enough to try a product if someone claims it will help them.

I'll be honest; in my (somewhat biased) opinion, it is wrong to tell a person that your product will heal them if you have no research to support the claim. You see, often, the companies behind these products will suggest that the product may help a certain condition. There's never any real research, and the testimonials can rarely be linked to an actual person.

Typically, the condition the product suggests it helps an illness with a huge patient base. I mean, what's the point of saying your magic smoothie mix helps a condition if the condition doesn't have a huge throng of suffering patients? The truth is that patients with complex medical histories should never start taking an unapproved mix of vitamins, minerals, and artificial coloring when their health is already hanging in the balance. Don't suggest they do unless you are the doctor directly managing their healthcare.

What's even more frustrating is that the marketing of these products places the blame on patients for their illness. I can't count how many times I've had my social media merchant friends post statuses that say things like, "When you get tired of spending money on doctor's visits, invest in your health by buying product X, Y, and Z." These posts are never directly pointed at me. More than likely, these posts are prewritten by the marketing team for their company. However, the fact remains that those selling these products are essentially telling patients that they have chosen to be sick by not buying their overpriced concoction.

So, please, as you embark on this journey of selling your new health product, I ask that you insert some kindness and grace into your marketing techniques. Don't prey on the ill. Instead, offer your product to those who show interest in it. Tell about the positive changes you've seen in your health; don't accuse others of not wanting to change simply because they won't buy whatever you're pushing. I am rooting for you. I love to support my friends on their entrepreneurial journeys. Heck, if you're selling leggings or a lipstick that won't make me look like I've been eating cherry popsicles, I'm buying. But, please, don't become another vulture. There are way too many of those out there.

Thanks for your time

Peace, love, and health.

CPSIA information can be obtained
at www.ICGtesting.com
Printed in the USA
BVHW031955141220
595705BV00017B/57